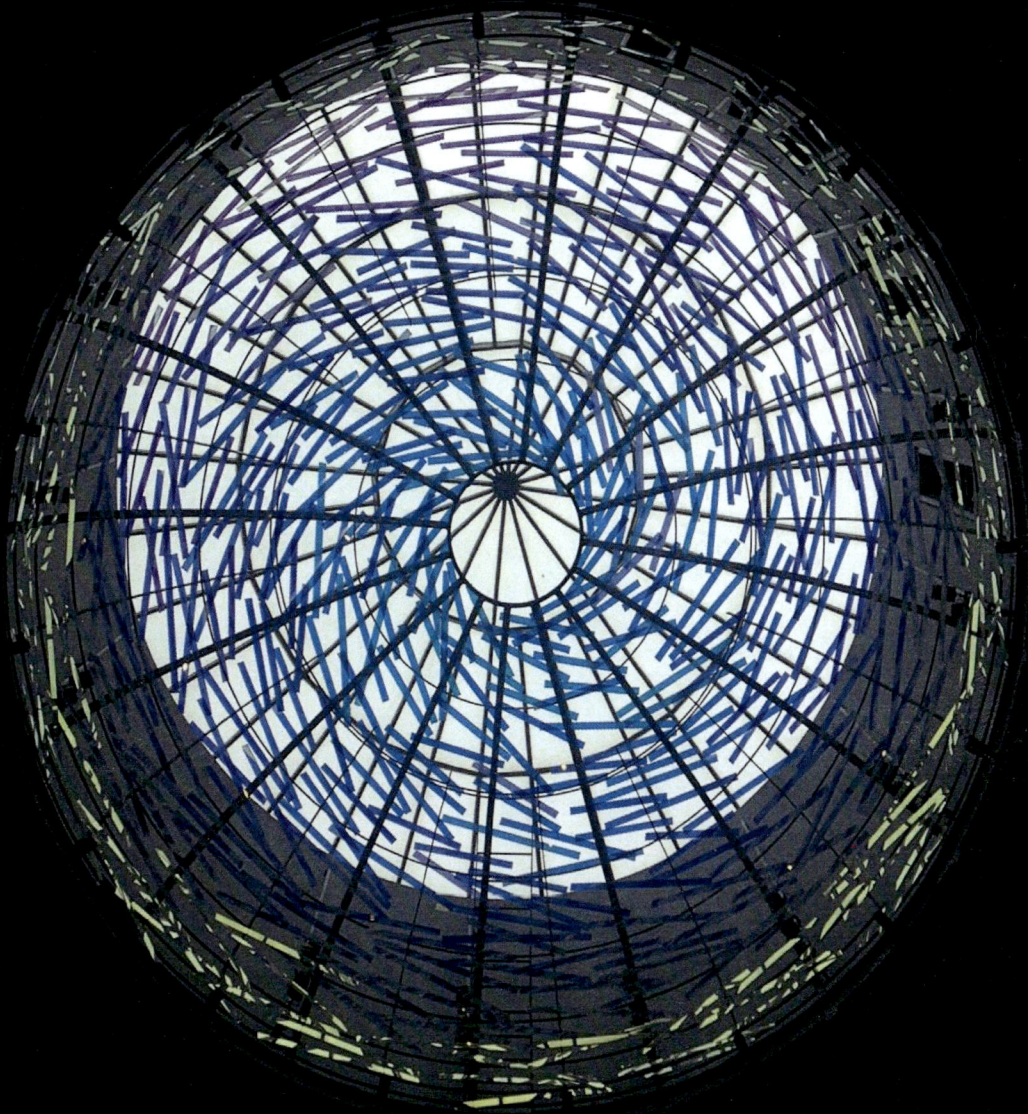

"If you can't fly then run, if you can't run then walk, if you can't walk then crawl, but whatever you do you have to keep moving forward."

**~ Martin Luther King Jr.**

"You never know how strong you are, until being strong is your only choice."

**~ Bob Marley.**

"Never let what you cannot do interfere with what you can do."

**~John Wooden**

"Believe in yourself and **DON'T GIVE UP!** Live with intention and die with intention. Take this life challenge and turn it into a life audit."

**~Michelle Lagos MBA**

### Photography:

**U P**
.
    Cover, insert, pages - 1, 25, 28, 30, 32, 39, 48, 52, 55 bio photo: **Michelle Lagos**

"Freedom" sculpture by Zenos Frudakis page 28.

### Graphic Design & Content:
**Michelle Lagos**

*This story is based on the true account of the inspirational near-death experience of Michelle Lagos to the best recount of facts available through medical documents, memory, and interviews.

THE

DEDICATION

OF THIS BOOK

IS SPLIT

TEN WAYS:


TO GOD – THANK YOU FOR A LIFETIME OF VISION AND PROTECTION

TO ERZSI – MY BEAUTIFUL DAUGHTER WHO CHOSE THE TITLE OF THE BOOK

TO ADAM NASH – MY TRUE FATHER

TO STEVEN – MY UNCLE/BROTHER/SOULMATE.

TO UNCLE NICK – THANK YOU FOR ALWAYS BELIEVING IN ME

TO THE INNER CIRCLE, FAMILY & FRIENDS - THAT SURROUND/ED ME   OXO

TO DR. JOHN ZURASKY – THANK YOU FOR SAVING MY LIFE AND MY SMILE!

TO DR. STERLING HODGSON – THANK YOU FOR SAVING MY LIFE AND HEARING!

TO DR. LISA YANASE – THANK YOU FOR CALLING THE 1ST SHOTS!

TO THE PROVIDENCE CARE STAFF – YOU'RE THE BEST!


*THANK YOU SO VERY MUCH FOR HELPING RESTORE MY LIFE!*

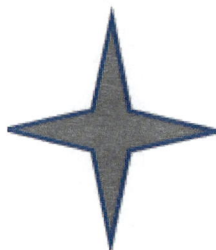

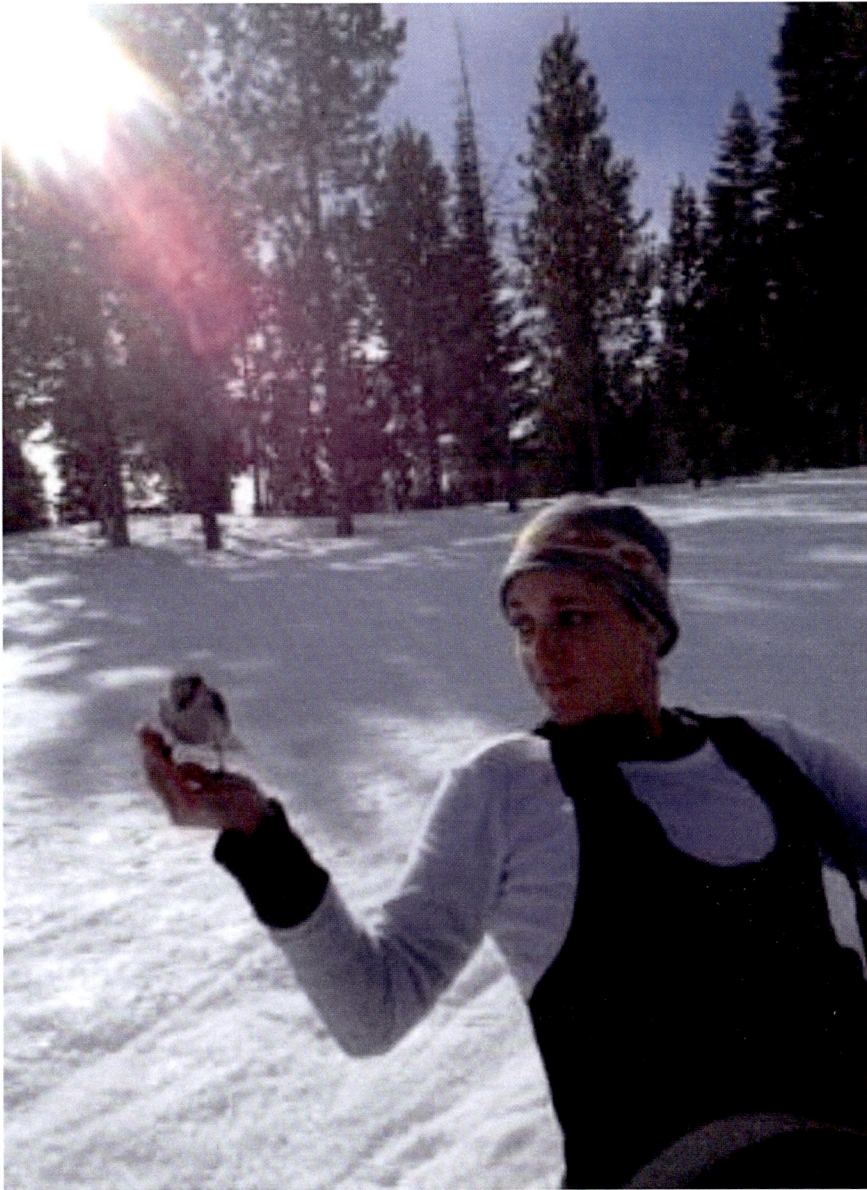

Bend, Oregon winter 2013

# CONTENTS

## REALITY POP!

## THE EXPERIENCE

>>>

### The Approach

This book was written with the consideration that there are typically 3 different kinds of learning styles that are learned best in combinations: auditory, visual, and kinesthetic, and also the intuitive that learns well with various textures.

This book also encourages the reader to ask the questions,

"Why am I here? What is my reason for living?"

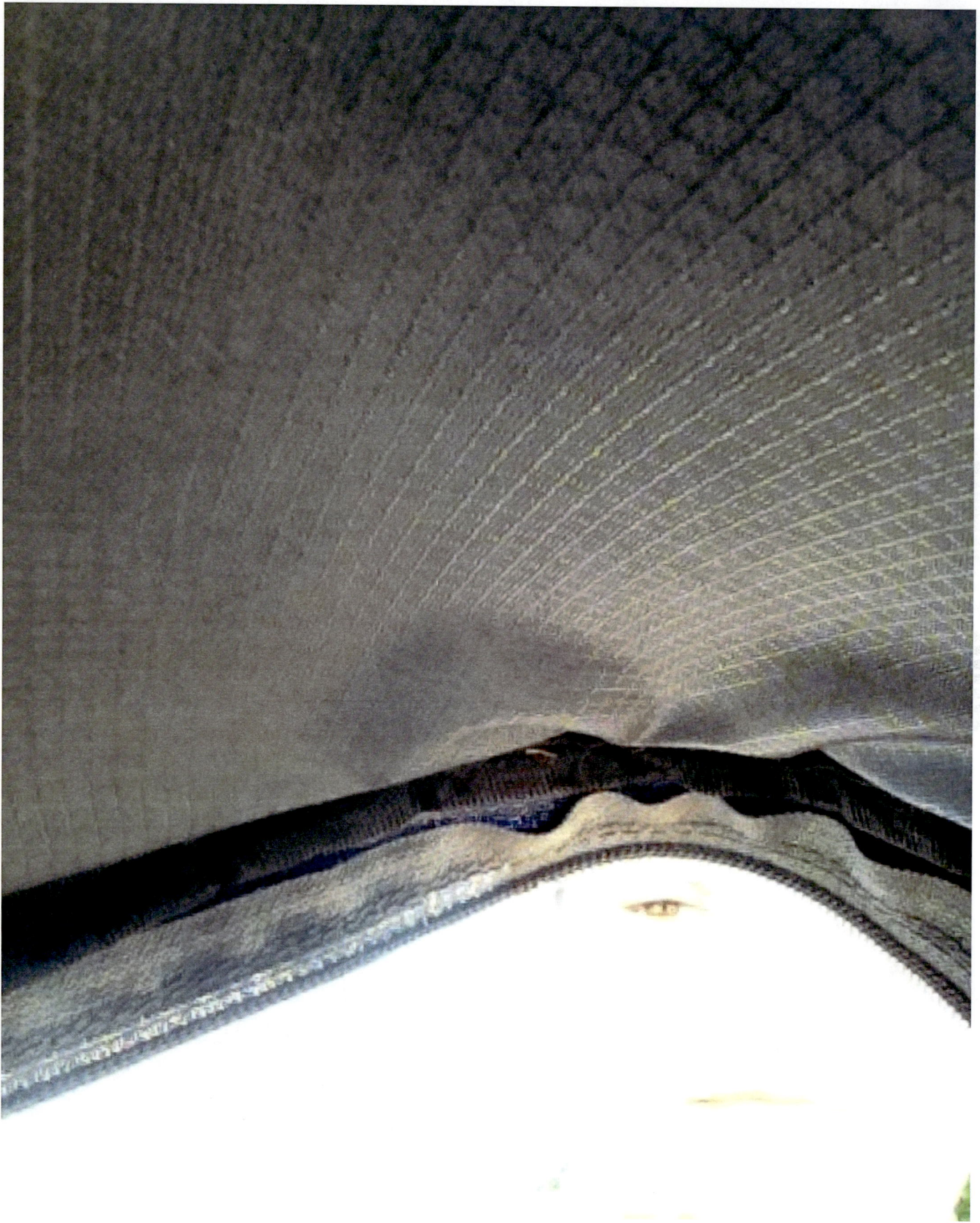

Running up a steep hill with a focused crowd, dirt being kicked into my nose and face, we rounded the corner of the first obstacle – a webbed tightrope structure over muddy water that you had to inch yourself across to keep balanced.

Next, the tire step-through obstacles and running over the top of muddy wrecked cars. Coming up over the slippery roofs you definitely got the **"I'm on top of the world"** feeling you always wanted, coupled with the **"I hope I'm not going to break anything today"** feeling.

Rounding the next corner the lake had big free floating logs we all climbed over, often throwing you off balance as your face plunged into the water with an occasional unknown body landing on top of you, or a muddy tennis shoe appearing near your face; holding your breath, or spitting out water, the wild challenge was still a flurry of **Fun**!

Without a second thought we ran off to push through to the muddy trenches to climb the muddy walls – determined and crossing fingers.

10 obstacles and 3 miles later we approached mud pools with barbed wire. As I inched along my stomach, military style, with my lips barely above the surface, I then jumped across a flame to the finish line, high on adrenaline and uninjured. **Victory**!

My wing Lori, and I, then jumped into big stagnant water pits with hundreds of other muddy racers, to shake off the caked mud layers with muddy water, later a hose removed more. Next, the 3 important B's were the primary source of enjoyment: Blanket, protein Bars and Beer, thus - **The Warrior's Lunch**

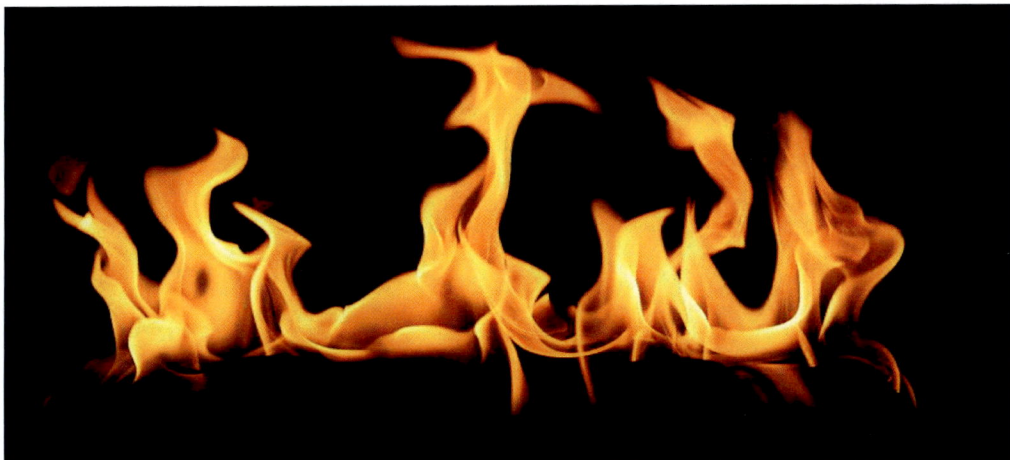

# Vision

# Focus

# Will

The next couple of weeks following the race I began hearing a watery swish sound in my right ear, similar to the sound effects of water entering into your ear during a shower, coupled with eardrum pressure, when I drove in elevated areas around Portland's West Hills.  Knowing that something was a bit off I checked in with the doctor and it was recommended I visit a specialist.  After the specialist visit it was decided I was grinding my teeth and it was recommended that I return to wearing a night guard when sleeping, practicing some relaxation techniques, and check back-in after vacation. Trusting the recommended specialist, who didn't test for an ear infection, I moved on with life and tried to ignore the pressure until the explosion.

Returning home from the San Juan Capistrano vacation on Nov. 8th, 2011 the plane began to circle **Portland, Oregon** with a breathtaking fall view of Mt. Hood.

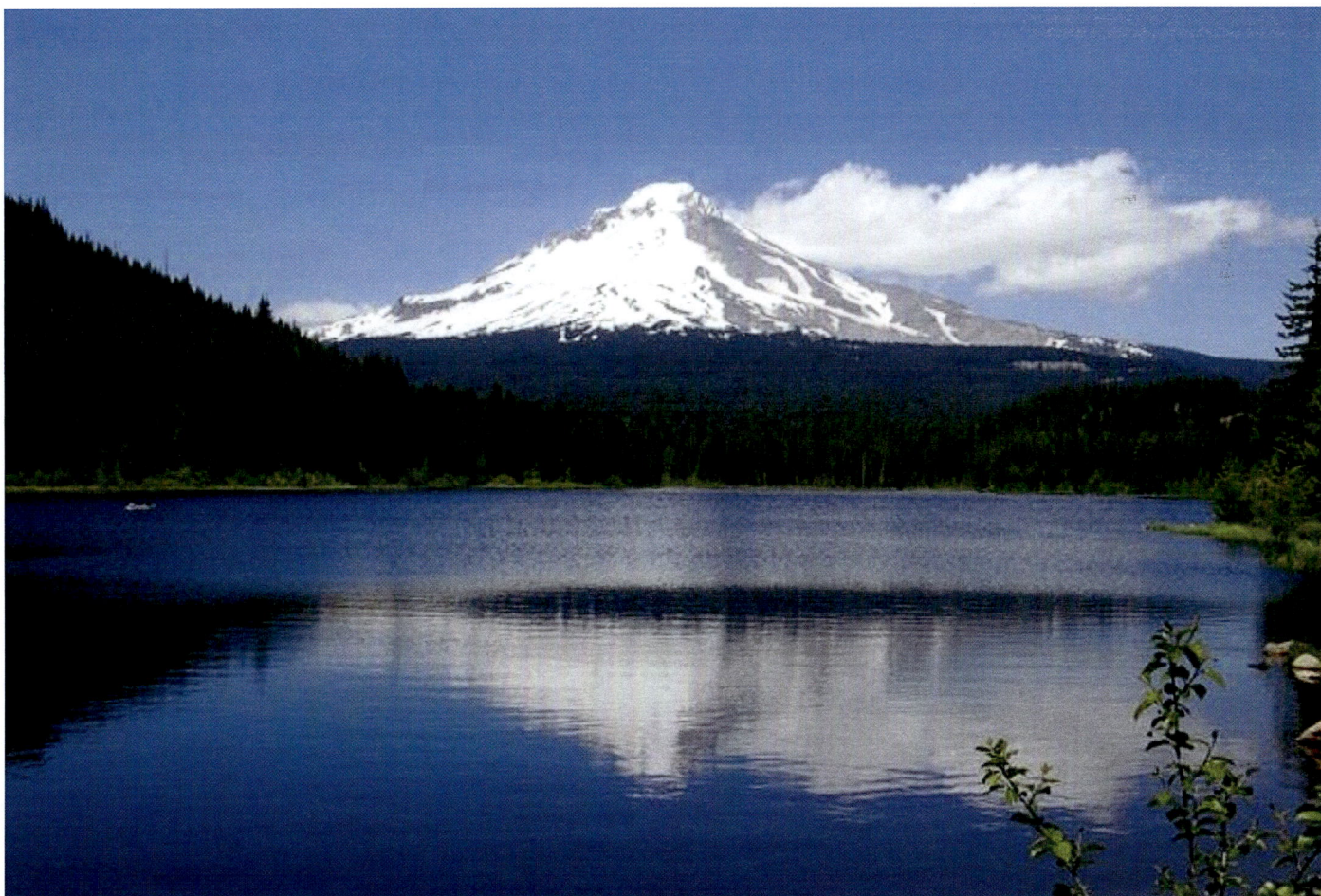

As the descend began the right ear that had that occasional swish and elevation sensitivity wasn't adjusting to the pressure changes and the inside pressure in the eardrum continued to intensify. Looking out the window, at the crystal blue sky full of white floating cumulus clouds (what seemed like a yard stick away from my window) no amount of jaw-clicking, yawning, or chewing helped the building pressure, unexpected sharp pain, or the loud clap of thunder that vibrated through my ear and head as my eardrum **exploded, exploded, exploded**…

In a very elevated state of pain, and not wanting to alarm my daughter, I silenced and focused, not discussing the situation with anyone as I calmly created a plan of action, in hopes of getting to solution as fast as possible. Upon landing I started placing tissue in my ear to absorb the blood and drainage, gathered our luggage, got the car, called my doctor, and headed straight for her office.

**Welcome Home.**

**Time to survive**.

At the appointment Dr. Le confirmed that the eardrum had ruptured and it simply needed time to heal and be monitored to determine if there was a need for surgery. For the time being antibiotics, pain killers, Advil, and home, was the recovery plan. Having never had surgery or a desire to take medication while leaving the pharmacy I took one of each, crossing fingers that the eardrum would heal quickly. After that first round of pills, I sat in the car Googling "ruptured eardrum stories" and trying to get an average on the amount of people that were able to move through the process non-surgically until I began to feel hints of the pain-killer-woo and decided it was time to get home before I got the light-headed giggles and the impaired "everything."

Arriving home a few minutes later, the person I was dating surprised me with flowers and a bag of groceries containing all that was needed for an amazing dinner. What a welcoming after such an **explosive** return.

Even with the desire to push aside the apparent circumstance and enjoy the welcoming date, later that afternoon I was flooded with a deep-seated feeling that something was severely wrong.

As the pain kept rapidly increasing, surpassing the pain relieving medication combinations, my calm bubble popped and I dropped to my knees in my bedroom and started crying. All I could see was a picture of my daughter in my minds' eye.  No, No, **NO**!  I was also concerned as the new and last term of my MBA program was beginning the following Monday, and I didn't want anything impeding my ability to finish it smoothly.

## Reason for Living:  Goals to support and accomplish – Still in love with life!

As the person I was dating came upstairs and found me processing, I found the pain, worry, and the moment of unplanned vulnerability especially uncomfortable, as I was used to being able to function with a large amount of reservation at that stage; and now life was just about to remind me of what faith, trust, and vulnerability truly was.

Reflecting, my core faith and strength that I had drawn from originated from being a youth that was an active high school member of the Eugene Free Methodist. The FMY group (Free Methodist Youth) were tightly webbed, took yearly missionary trips to Mexico, and had a focus on giving back, mentorship, and "doing to others as you would want done to you" while playing a LOT!  These core desires/philosophies moved on with me as I explored my spirituality as an adult, and had a deep-seated desire to educate and draw in wisdom from multiple sources and cultures.  Later, still being Christ-centric, but liberal, I began to embrace positive resources that were also useful for both the mental/physical/spiritual aspects of life such as the wisdom of :

**Zen Buddhism:**  Meditation, visualization, chanting, and sensory expansion exercises.
**Yoga**:  Deep breathing, balancing, chakra energy work while gaining the extraordinary strength and flexibility of  both vinyasa yoga in the spring/summer/fall and bikram yoga in the winter.
**Reiki:**  1st and 2nd degree, which is hand energy healing work, much akin to  the sensations that I felt as a youth when we would pray and lay our hands on each other.

**Cun Tao Martial Arts**:  Which taught me how to use focus and will to strengthen and control the body while working with energy and fighting techniques.

And lastly, I found jogging, trail running, and hiking all meditation in motion and found myself often feeling the closest to God when I was standing on top of a mountain looking at nature, and the vast beauty of Oregon, without the words and thoughts of someone else - but simply in the beauty of silence.

Later that night, in a hazed elevated level of pain, I wondered downstairs, took a bath, and laid down on the floor of my daughter's bedroom and went back to sleep. That's all I remember until a week later, when I briefly woke up in ICU surrounded by family and close friends.

The next morning I was found in my daughter's bedroom speaking incoherently with a high fever; an ambulance was then called, and I was swiftly whisked away to the SE Providence ICU. There it was determined that I had rapid brain swelling with bacterial meningitis that had entered in through my ruptured eardrum, as the inner ear infection passed through the barriers. To try to combat the brain swelling a tube was inserted into my brain and IVs with large doses of fluids, antibiotics, steroids, and blood thinners were given.

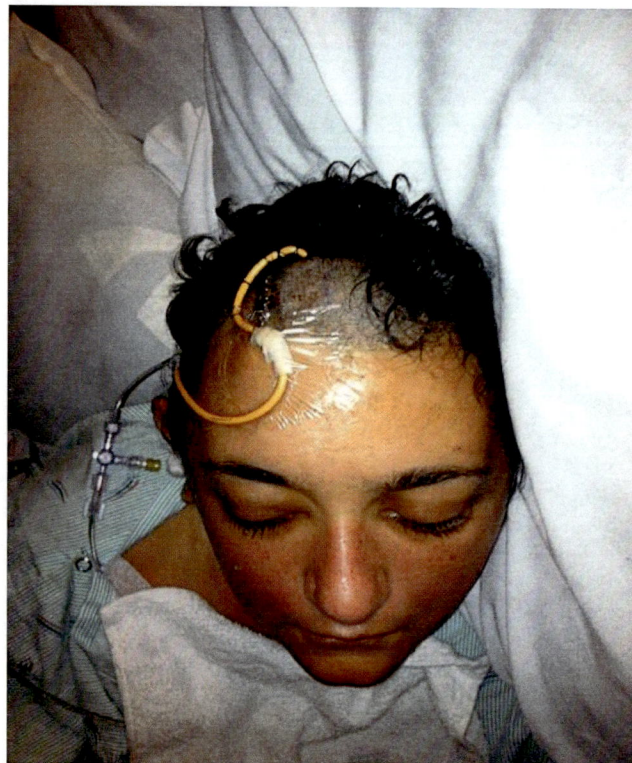

As the recovery in ICU was moving slower than hoped Dr. Sterling Hodgson, Otolaryngologist (medical specialty concerned with the ear, nose, and throat) was called in to evaluate the ruptured eardrum and canal, and discovered that the inner ear explosion had caused the infection to spread into the mastoid air cells, which are the cells that sit in a hollow space in the skull, behind the ear. To secure that the infection didn't continue to spread throughout even more bone, that would also have to be removed, a mastoidectomy was performed.  This successful surgery removed the infected air cell bone areas behind the ear, which then left a two-inch concave area with the ear canal being fully drained.

Even though I had either temporary or permanent facial nerve paralysis, I had essentially lost the ability to blink my left eye independently, without the assistance of the other eye, nor smile as the left side of my face laid mostly inactive like a mini-mudslide.

It was determined that if the surgery hadn't been performed, with the fast spreading infection and brain swelling, there would've been **no** chance of survival. This was one of the first times my family was warned I may not survive the process.  **"It would be a strong battle to fight."**

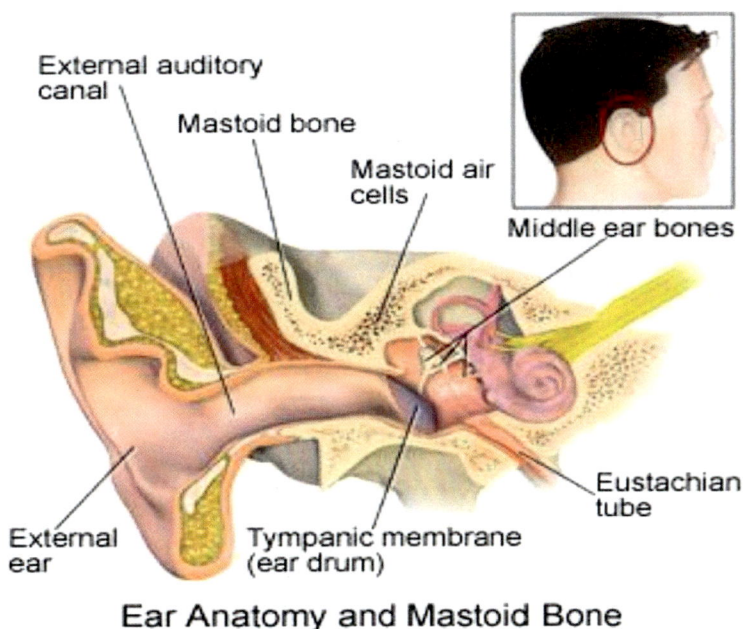

Ear Anatomy and Mastoid Bone

**"Be strong and courageous. Do not be afraid or terrified... your God goes with you;" Deuteronomy 31:6**

As the weeks continued the chances of survival increased as I was stabilizing, the brain swelling reduced, and the infection was controlled.

The first time I awoke for a period longer than 10 minutes it occurred in the middle of the night, in my private recovery room. At that time, I was having visions of a view of the SW Portland hills, that I used to see looking out the windows in my ceramics and life drawing classes (during my bachelor's courses) and I started reviewing prior life decisions and questioning them. After hours of staring at the window and wall reflecting, I came to conclusion that I was at complete peace with my core life decisions but had the desire to reconnect with a handful of friends/mentors from childhood, and the early 20s, as well as move forward with the high-risk youth volunteerism that I had grown so passionate about. As those visions began to fade away there was a white board in front of me with my uncle Steven's name and number, and the person I was dating's name and number, in **green**. As the period of contemplation extended I became alarmed after being alone for so long, and was relieved when the nurse came in and I was able to ask if she'd let me use her cellphone. The nurse kindly touched my hand, gave me her cellphone, and told me to use it as long as I wanted… Yes, this is the extraordinary care and kindness I continued to receive, as well as my family, during this entire experience.

As the days passed family and friends came every day with tasty treats, photos, smiles, hugs, and touch therapy like massage, foot rubs, reiki, and even toenail painting, as the Providence staff kindly honored our wishes and allowed my family to be present with me as many hours as we preferred, as well as let as many friends join us as the family decided was best day-by-day. This open atmosphere gave me a great sense of comfort and security as I felt surrounded by the people I loved, opposed to feeling lonely and isolated. It was good reminder to always see why you're fighting and why you'll **NEVER** stop while asking the important self-questions, **"Why am I here? What is my reason for living?"**

At this stage I was calmly fighting with steroids that had blown my body up to 250+ lbs. and I was grateful for the simple things, like laughter and cold water. Oh, and the relative that thought he knew how to do the moonwalk for a couple of seconds here and there.

Regardless, when I looked down at my hands, feet, or my face in the mirror, I had morphed into a person I didn't recognize and it silently pained me. Where I had at one time did some plus-size modeling, I wondered in those moments, if I would even be able to smile again much less look like/be a fraction of me again.

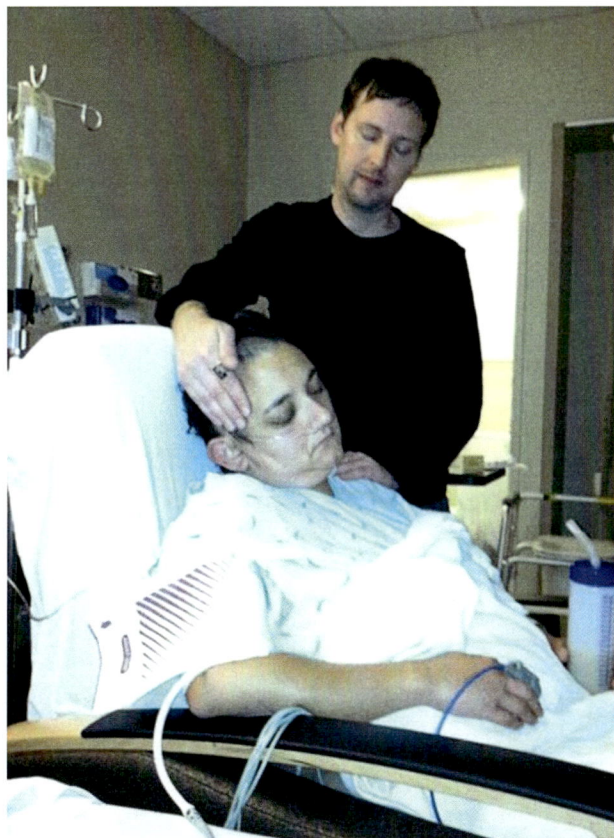

As more of my fears continued I wondered if I would ever have my independence again, be able to creatively/professionally produce on the level I was used too, be the capable and effective mother I had planned to be, date, or enjoy the level of freedom/play/adventure that I use as my main enjoyment of life and my primary coping tool. The feelings of worry were unsolvable and unable to help support the determination and focus I needed to push the healing forward, so I found that it was best to ignore that there would be any other outcome than **complete** recovery. Sheer spiritual focus and faith of the visions I saw of the future was a tremendous help.

## Reason for Living: Goals to support and accomplish – Still in love with life!

Behind the scenes relatives were being told that it may take up to 3 years for me to recover, partially or fully, and that the process could take many twists and turns.

So, it wasn't a surprise that occasionally during the initial healing process I would get inspired, and manically repeat ideas (often positive-focused) in a looping form, and at other times when I was done with items, toss them across the room, and then sometimes obsess about their location.

Of course, with all fine-motor skills challenged, I still retained the ability to use the cellphone and navigate Facebook, as no amount of trauma seems to pull most people too far away from their I-Phone, as was also my truth. The phone was one of my main forms of entertainment, giving me the ability to stay connected outside of the confines of the room.

To everyone's surprise, slowly the throwing became a short toss to a desired vicinity, and my ability to shorten the passionate focused loops occurred. Now, it became a waiting game to see how many of my motor skills would be regained as well… until Thanksgiving Day.

On Thanksgiving afternoon the uncles rounded the corner with smiles and a full Thanksgiving feast that included homemade cranberry sauce, turkey, mashed potatoes and gravy, bourbon mushroom soup, salad, chocolates, and a fragrant pumpkin pie with freshly whipped cream. My family loves to cook and find ways to celebrate. So, on this day, being the first holiday of the season, everyone wanted to celebrate the healing progress as all signs of the infection being gone was confirmed, the brain swelling reduced to normal, and the ear canal and air cell areas were healing well. I was also staying awake and interactive for longer periods of time with short periods of reading and writing. All was grateful to celebrate being out of woods!

As the day continued, and more family and extended family stopped in for a visit, a gradual but raging headache began that eventually caused me to hold my head, grimacing with my eyes closed. In an large amount of pressure pain and too intense to cry, I kept on repeating, **"It hurts too much. Too much."** Alarmed and feeling helpless my uncle Steven sensed the emergency and when the nurse arrived into the room she did a quick evaluation and ordered an MRI (Magnetic Resonance Imaging).

Soon after my neurologist, Dr. John Zurasky, arrived from his holiday evening to review the MRI and deliver the fateful news to family in the hallway. Showing the shaded areas on the scan to family, John gave his sincere regrets as he announced that I had a bilateral hemorrhage (both sides of my brain were heavily bleeding) and they had 30 minutes to say goodbye, as my memory would soon be permanently gone, and I would be dying sometime that evening.

The shock and disbelief kept the small group discussing it. "What are the chances she can make it?" Steven inquired. Dr. Zurasky sadly responded, "I'm sorry Steven, people don't make it through this. At this point you wouldn't want her too, as there's a good chance she'd be a vegetable for the rest of her life." Steven stared at Dr. Zurasky with the feeling that his jaw just hit his chest and his legs were buckling. Unable to move Steven stood there frozen until Dr. Zurasky stopped the conversation and announced. "Time is running out. You need to get her to the ICU room and say your goodbyes."

Pushing me from the recovery room to the ICU room, the family/extended family discussions continued, as I laid there hearing everything heavily medicated, I slightly, but very determined raised my head and firmly said, **"I'm not going anywhere!"** As they continued talking and crying, I instinctually knew it was time to focus and block them out, using the same techniques I learned in meditation and martial arts. So I lowered my head, closed my eyes, and visualized the two areas in my brain that were bleeding and pictured healing white light where the bleeding was occurring. It's as if I willed the leaking blood to turn off like a faucet; and in minds' eye I saw it occur. It seemed that God/Universe and I grabbed a handle on that one together.

**Thank you. Thank you. I'm not going anywhere! ...**

Soon all the nurses that had cared for me began to enter my ICU room crying, as my family surrounded my head. As Uncle Steven began to explain the results to the rest of the family, I silenced outwardly but with my inside soul voice I just kept saying, **"Thank you"** before falling asleep peacefully. At this time all those around me thought these were my last moments. Trying to reach for each other and be philosophical, the family sat together as the 30 minutes passed. 2 hours passed. 3 hours passed and I did not. On the 3rd hour another MRI was ordered and much to everyone's surprise, but just as I saw it, the bleeding had **STOPPED**.

Yes, miracles do exist. Soon after family was encouraged to go home and rest as the next day could bring any surprise. Exiting that evening, many were still in a state of disbelief as "People don't survive this," and "How can she keep going on fighting like this?" Gratefully from this point forward there were no setbacks and the healing process continued rapidly. Still it was never fast enough for me, as I wanted my complete independence back, at such a core level, that with every inch of progress there was another inch of impatience to want the process to move along at lightning speed. Even though I innately was grateful and polite to all I came into contact with, I was tired of being touched, poked into, and arranged. I simply wanted to take a run in the woods, go listen to a live band, eat some amazing food in one of our cultural rich neighborhoods, and get lost at will.

As the days moved forward I was released back to my recovery room and much of the same healing cycle that occurred the last time continued again but with reading, regular visits with my daughter, and a better handle on working with utensils and writing. At this period of recovery, family was warned that I may or may not ever be able to work again or return to finish the Master's but I most certainly would not be a vegetable and would be functioning on at least a base level. With much planning behind the scenes happening, family chose not to disclose this information to me so I could better focus on healing.

During this period friends and family came together (like the last round of recovery) and created visiting shifts and teamed together with various strengths and skillsets to handle any needs that arose, in or out of the hospital.

The event had bonded everyone and given them a new reality on the importance of appreciating life and the care they would desire if they had a medical emergency occur.

The inner circle team, at one point, decided it was time to begin lightening the air in the recovery room and started having various ethnic meals brought in with the I-Phone speaker attachment for our entertainment pleasure. This added lively moments with fingers snapping, in the well-decorated room with a nice SE view, surrounded in photos, cards, poems, and flowers, but that modeling shot still sat across the room staring at me… Being a spirited Italian and Cajun-French woman it was decided that someday there needed to be a dance floor to twirl around on soon, but for now there just wasn't another option, so the room would do perfectly.

**"If you can't fly then run (or dance), if you can't run (or dance) then walk, if you can't walk then crawl, but whatever you have to do to keep moving forward**." **Martin Luther King Jr**.

With independence being the primary desire, during one visit with family, I looked over at the restroom and had the "I want to wash my own face and use the bathroom on my own" feeling, so I ripped my IV out of my way and charged into the bathroom. Before the alarmed family could reach me I had already shut the door and was having a moment of "restroom solace" with a strong look of "**Don't**" when the door was reopened. As much as this particular instance struck a moment of stress in many, it was actually a great turning point and a celebration of strength as we're designed to **Get Back UP** and fight for survival when you have -

## Goals to support and accomplish – Still in love with life!

Yes, **DO** and **DON'T** were an important focus with **CAN** and **WILL.** Determined, with an occasional freedom flare-up such as this, the physical therapist began coming in and taking me for regular walks and yoga stretches, as I was used to being very active and as I strengthened, my auto-pilot was being triggered. Safe independence was the perfect springboard to help encourage the new zoom.

Much to the care staffs surprise my motor and cognitive skills began restoring quickly and in the second week of December it was decided that if healing remained on the same trajectory, I would be returning home for Christmas on December 20th. And December 20th it was.

Before leaving the hospital Dr. John Zurasky and I had a memorable one-on-one talk where he encouraged me to keep focusing on healing and relaxing enough to let the process continue safely (as he knew I was willful and driven to move it **ALL** forward as quick as humanly, or possibly not humanly possible), allow my family to help me, rest, and not to worry that I was on 6 medications and would need some homecare for a period of time. I thanked him for helping save my life as he's truly a strong, caring, one-of-kind person. I also shared my same goals/focuses during the conversation with a strong desire to first get off of every medication, cleanse, learn how to run again, and learn how to wink and smile at anyone I wanted too. We both laughed as John said, "Michelle, I know you will. I just know it.

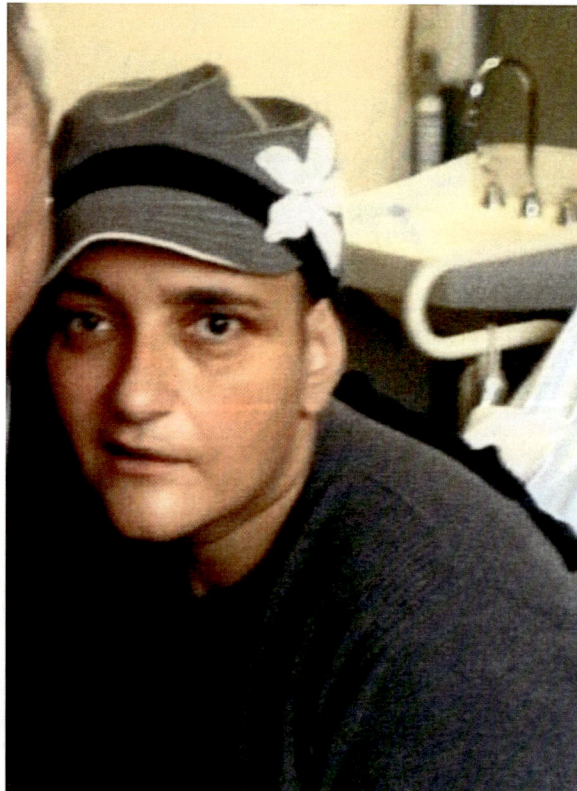

**Packing to leave the hospital.**

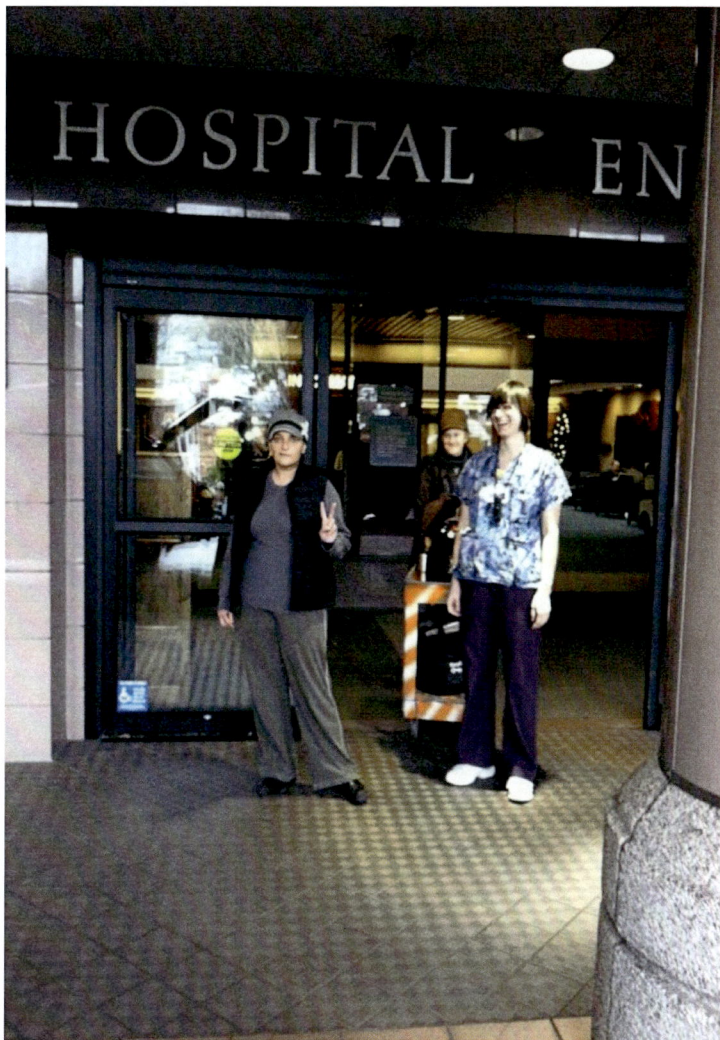

Hugging the nurses and leaving the hospital.

## Victory!

Crossing another finish line, I'm homeward bound.

It was time to train, pray, and **PLAY**!

**Reason for Living**: Goals to support and accomplish – Still in love with life!

Returning home was nothing short of a sigh of relief and a time to focus on **The Recovery Plan** I had made as the next leg of the journey it was time for me to take control of my healthcare and move forward with many athletic, spiritual, and Eastern medicine practices I'd used to completely recover from two intense car accidents and a time of unhealthy obesity in the past.

**Welcome Home**

*When was a time you went through a healing?  What was your **Recovery Plan**?  Did it Work?  What did you do?  Reflect and write all that you remember.*

_____

_____

_____

_____

_____

_____

_____

_____

_____

_____

_____

_____

_____

_____

_____

_____

_____

_____

_____

_____

_____

_____

*Share your Recovery Plan & Experience with me at **GetBackUP-Book.com***

*When did you feel most empowered?  When did you the feel safest?*

_____

_____

_____

_____

_____

_____

_____

_____

_____

_____

_____

_____

_____

_____

_____

_____

_____

_____

_____

_____

_____

_____

_____

Share your thoughts with me at **GetBackUP Book.com** and
**https://www.facebook.com/getbackup2015**

One of the greatest lessons of strength I learned through the near death experiences at the hospital, that also became a great life asset during the healing period and life forward, was the ability to completely focus inward as needed, and not absorb the fears and thoughts of others as absolute truth. This applied to the healing process, as I continued to move at super speed, which was often a surprise and stressful for those around me; as my focus stayed forward from conscious effort but also because medications were wisely given to me to block sections of the trauma memories that I simply didn't need to think and focus on.

In reflection, please write your thoughts on the recovery and support caregivers could use for good self-care during moments such as these.

_____

_____

_____

_____

_____

_____

_____

_____

_____

_____

Share your thoughts with me at *GetBackUP-Book.com*

# The Daily Recovery Plan

- Eat only organic food – the body was filtering enough chemicals and needed nutrient rich, non-poisonous options.

  - **Recommendations**: Shop at local farmer's markets - **http://www.localharvest.org/farmers-markets/list?l=M.**
  - **More advice on saving $:** **http://www.ourordinarylife.com/2011/01/buying-organic-foods-at-a-discount-free-organic-food-coupons/**
  - **http://moneysavingmom.com/2012/03/how-to-afford-organic-foods-on-a-budget.html**
  - **Find Community Supported Agriculture Groups near you** - **https://www.biodynamics.com/content/community-supported-agriculture-introduction-csa**
  - **National Co-op Directory** **http://www.coopdirectory.org/directory.htm**
  - **Google – Organic food delivery**

- Juice and eat as many fruits and vegetables as possible.

  - **Recommendation:** Gather organic recipes and coupons online - **http://foodbabe.com/recipe-rendezvous/.**
  - **Juicing – http://www.today.com/food/clean-green-healthy-juice-recipes-make-blender-t20421**
  - **Juicing - http://www.today.com/food/clean-green-healthy-juice-recipes-make-blender-t20421**
  - **Raw Salads - http://www.choosingraw.com/recipes/salads/**
  - **Raw Salads - http://www.rawguru.com/raw-food-recipes/**
  - **Super Salads -** **https://www.thehealthychef.com/category/recipes/super-salads/**

- Drink primarily distilled water.

- Do gentle yoga stretching every day, for even 15 minutes and build-up to an hour and a weekly session with an in-house instructor.

    - **Recommendation**: Watch this video and stay inspired: **https://www.youtube.com/watch?v=qX9FSZJu448**

- Build up the walking time – 10, 15, 20, 30 minutes.  At 30 minutes jog for 5, 10, 15, 20 minutes. The cardio felt like soaring while increasing fresh oxygen and blood flow to my body and brain.

    - **Why Running is good for your brain, health, and circulation: https://www.psychologytoday.com/blog/neuronarrative/201 009/why-running-is-incredible-medicine-your-brain**
    - **http://www.medicaldaily.com/run-your-life-6-health-benefits-running-just-5-minutes-every-day-322050**
    - **https://experiencelife.com/article/how-exercise-heals/**
    - **http://med.stanford.edu/news/all-news/2008/08/running-slows-the-aging-clock-stanford-researchers-find.html**

- Rest and sleep immediately as needed.  Don't fight it. Feel like you have permission to ask for the care you need.

    - **Recommended: http://www.dailymail.co.uk/health/article-90598/What-happens-body-youre-asleep.html**
    - **http://www.huffingtonpost.com/maria-rodale/the-healing-nature-of-sle_b_4651358.html**

- Pray often, be grateful, and thank God and the universe, etc. for every day.

- **Recommended:**
  http://www.forbes.com/sites/amymorin/2014/11/23/7-scientifically-proven-benefits-of-gratitude-that-will-motivate-you-to-give-thanks-year-round/

- **10-15 minutes** of deep-breathing.

  - **Recommended:** http://www.health.harvard.edu/mind-and-mood/relaxation-techniques-breath-control-helps-quell-errant-stress-response
  - **Breathing Techniques:** https://chopra.com/ccl/breathing-for-life-the-mind-body-healing-benefits-of-pranayama
  - **Mind/Body Connecting:**
    http://my.clevelandclinic.org/services/heart/prevention/emotional-health/stress-relaxation/mind-body-exercises

- Meditate and visualize future accomplishments – Mine was running a 5K that winter, smiling, winking, dancing, graduating with my **MBA** and volunteering.

  - **Recommended:**
    https://www.psychologytoday.com/blog/flourish/200912/seeing-is-believing-the-power-visualization
  - **Miracle story:** http://www.huffingtonpost.com/russell-bishop/miracles-power-of-visualization-_b_1128113.html
  -

- Read, do crosswords, and write at least a paragraph of anything. It was time to get the snappy brain back into full-force.

  - **Recommended:** http://www.brainhq.com/why-brainhq/brain-training-your-way/12-benefits-of-brain-fitness

23

- Massage, acupuncture, and neuro-feedback weekly.

    - **Benefits of Massage:** http://www.mayoclinic.org/healthy-lifestyle/stress-management/in-depth/massage/art-20045743
    - http://www.oprah.com/health/The-Health-Benefits-of-Massage
    - **Benefits of Acupuncture:** http://www.medicalnewstoday.com/articles/156488.php
    - **Benefits of Neuro-feedback:** http://betterbrainsinc.com/faq.htm

- Facial and winking exercises and facial pressure point work and massage.

    - **Recommendation: Facial Paralysis and Bells Palsy exercise videos on You Tube.**

- Laugh and play as often as possible!

    - **Recommendation:** http://www.realsimple.com/health/preventative-health/health-benefits-play
    - http://psychcentral.com/blog/archives/2012/11/15/the-importance-of-play-for-adults/

- Practice positive self-talk and have HOPE and a Can DO attitude!

    - **Recommendation: Read the Power of Positive Thinking**
    - http://www.healthy-holistic-living.com/power-of-positive-thinking.html

- **http://consumer.healthday.com/encyclopedia/holistic-medicine-25/holistic-medicine-news-383/positive-psychology-a-new-approach-to-mental-health-648414.html- Check out the Positivity in Action List.**
- **http://www.movemequotes.com/top-15-power-of-positive-thinking-quotes/**

**Results:** A rapid recovery that included an quick increase in energy, strength, balance, concentration, peace of mind, confidence, and hope.

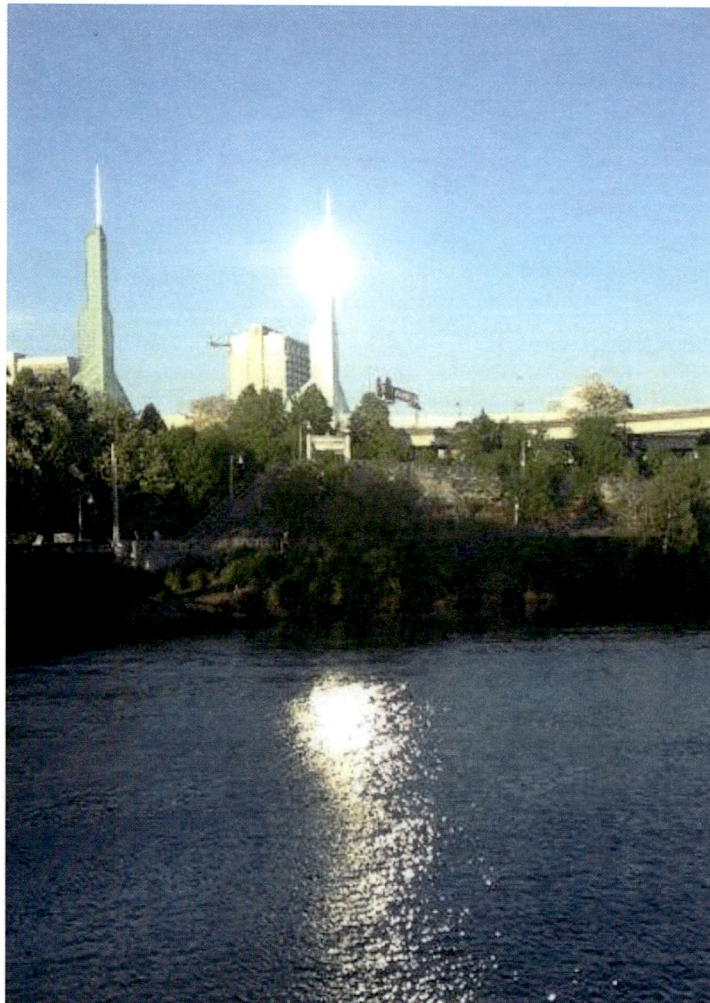

# What are your thoughts after you stare here?

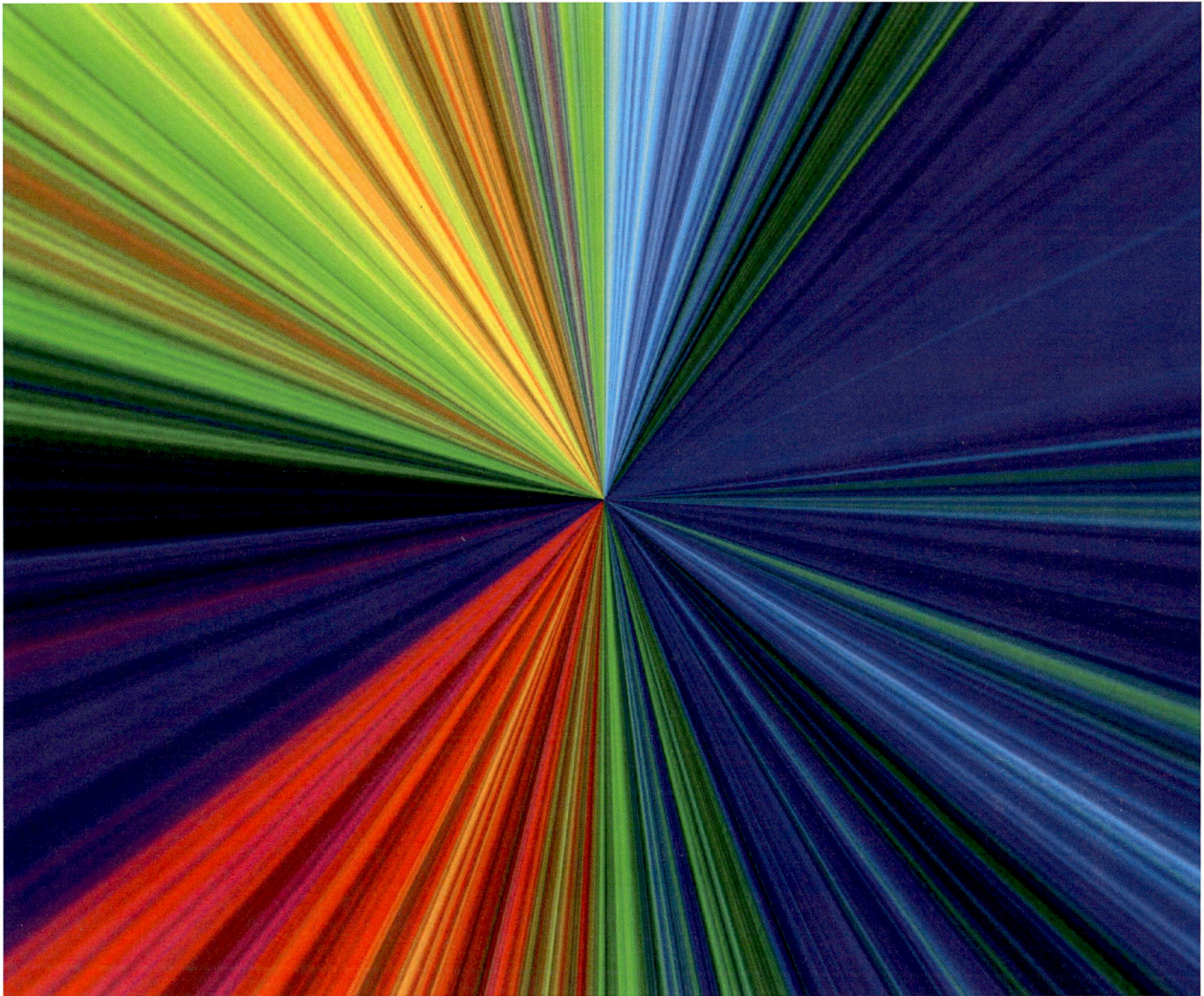

_____
_____
_____
_____
_____
_____
_____
_____
_____

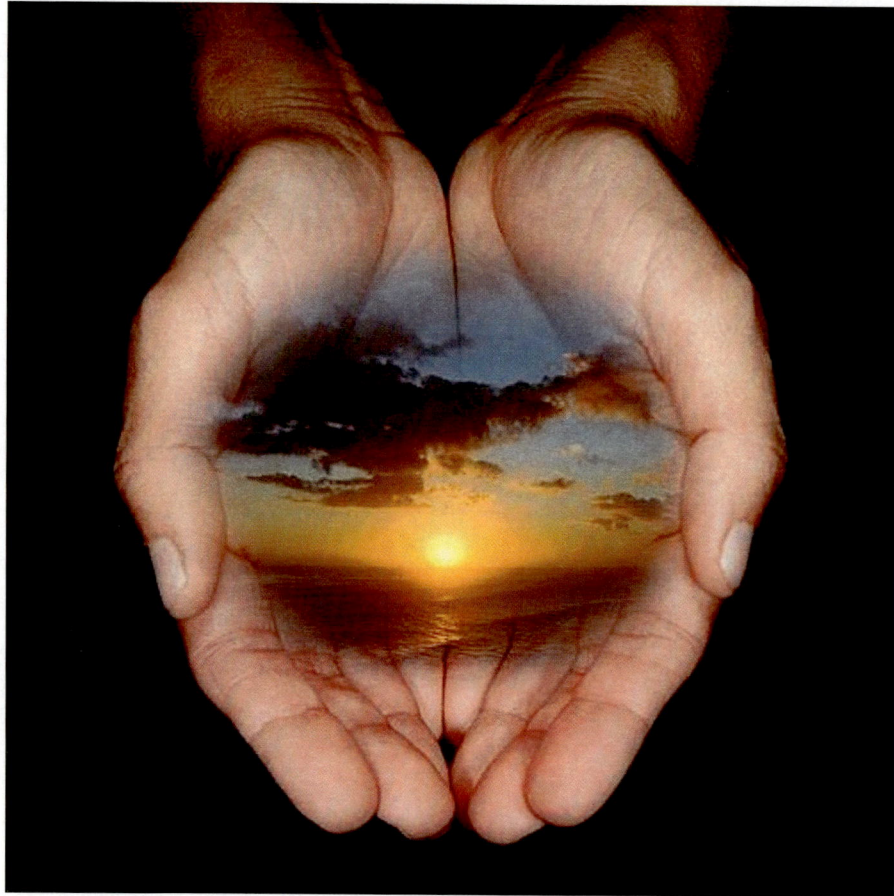

Write the ways you contribute to the positive both **small** and **large**. Every act of simple kindness matters.

_____

_____

_____

_____

_____

Share your thoughts with me  at  *GetBackUP-Book.com* and
https://www.facebook.com/getbackup2015

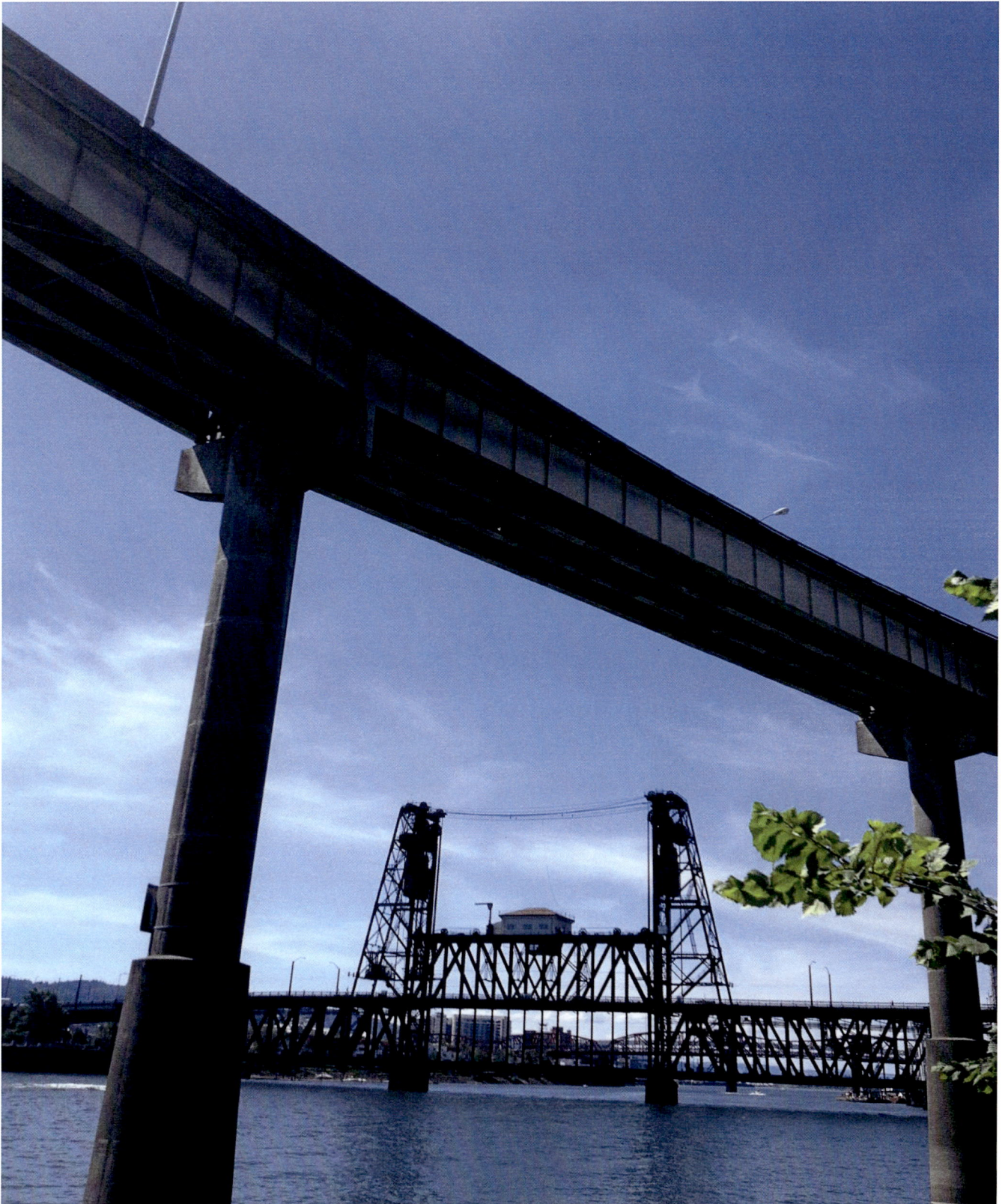

Commit to your passion in the world

and don't be derailed...

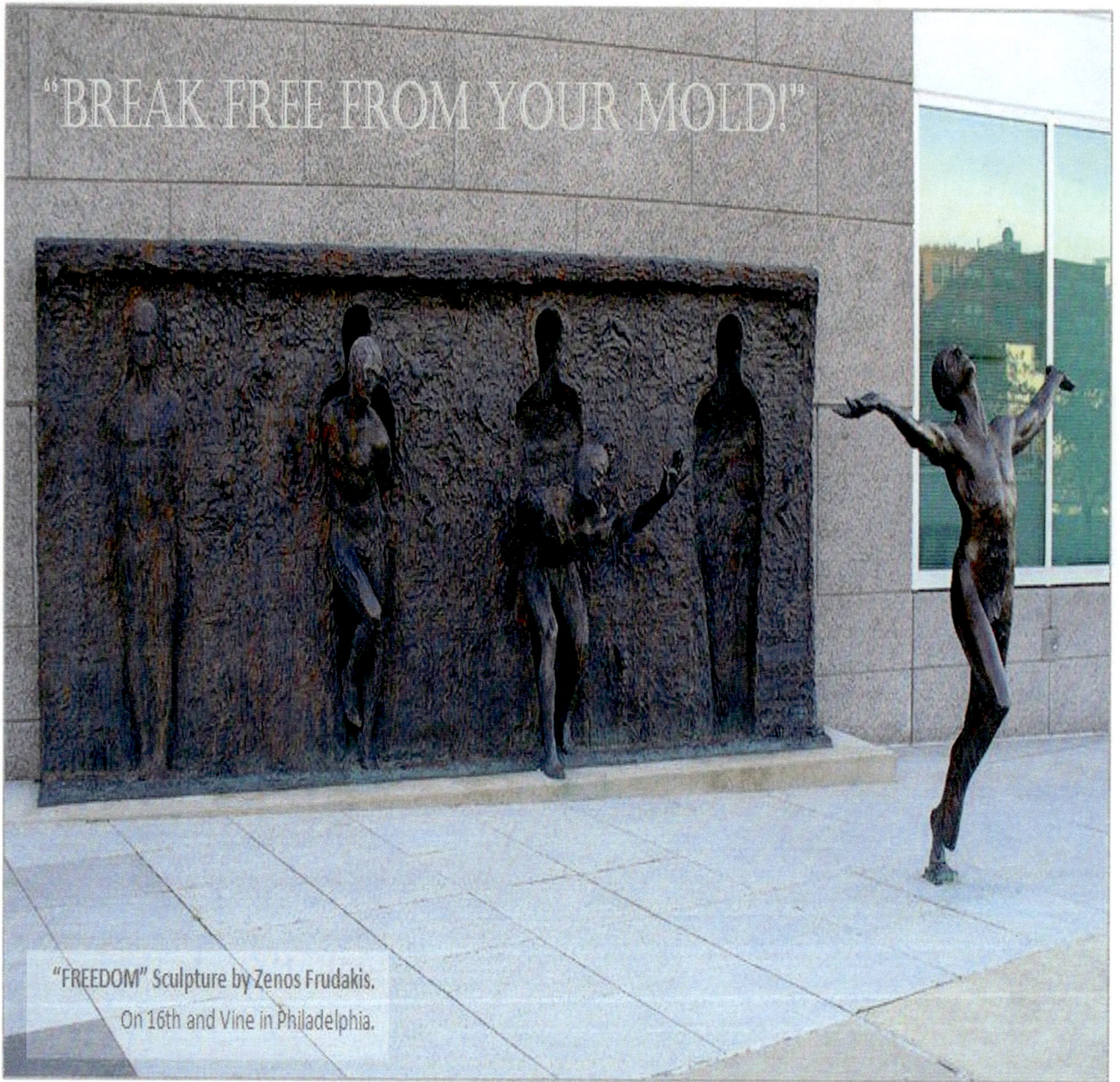

"BREAK FREE FROM YOUR MOLD!"

"FREEDOM" Sculpture by Zenos Frudakis.
On 16th and Vine in Philadelphia.

Every day is a gift!

Returning to a clean home 5.5 weeks later and also to a large bouquet of flowers, a house full of my favorite foods, all the bills paid, all the medical paperwork in order, with Christmas presents placed under the tree for my daughter, and myself, was just a **WOW**! My friends and family were SO thoughtful, SO protective, and SO welcoming that it shined even brighter that I was SO fortunate. Even with the paralysis face, I was simply grateful to be **FREE.** Now the most important step was to **move into action** and put the recovery plan into full effect with the same focus I used to stop the bleeding, walk again, talk again, and even throw an unwanted item across the room with fingers snapping as needed.

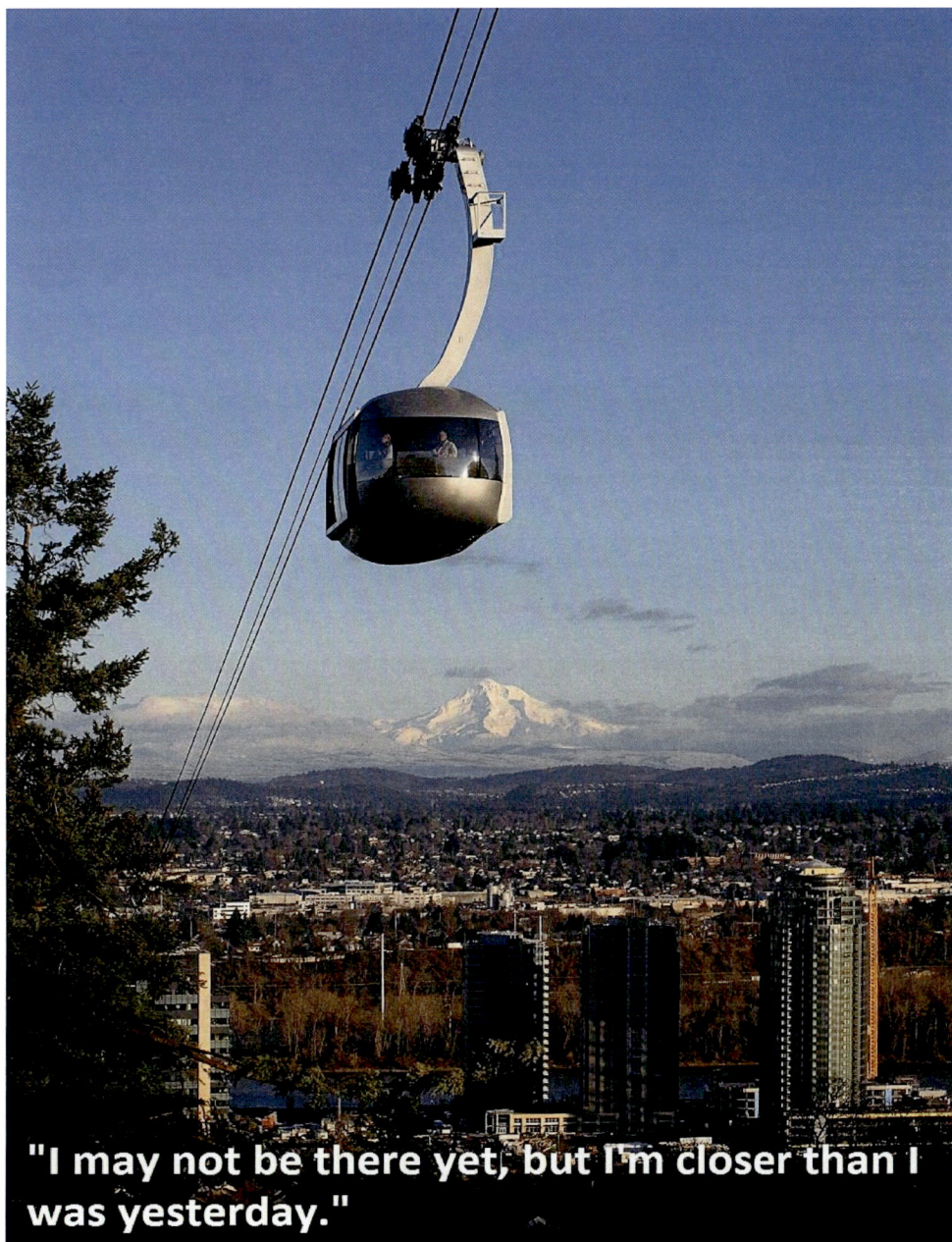

"I may not be there yet, but I'm closer than I was yesterday."

The next month I moved forward with the recovery plan I had created and was pleased with the rapid results. It was thrilling to go from 3 short naps a day to 1. Begin walking 10 minutes slowly to 20 minutes quickly, and jog 4 minutes too. Sometimes mid-day into the evening, after my facial muscles warmed up, I could almost get my left eye to wink independently and get the corner of my mouth to move upward a hint more. Yoga was also a pleasure as it was nice to be able to move into deep positions again, and hold them for long periods, as I had been practicing for 13 years prior, and I still find the pretzel-time very relaxing and enjoy staying flexible while contemplating, **"Why am I here? What is my reason for living?"**

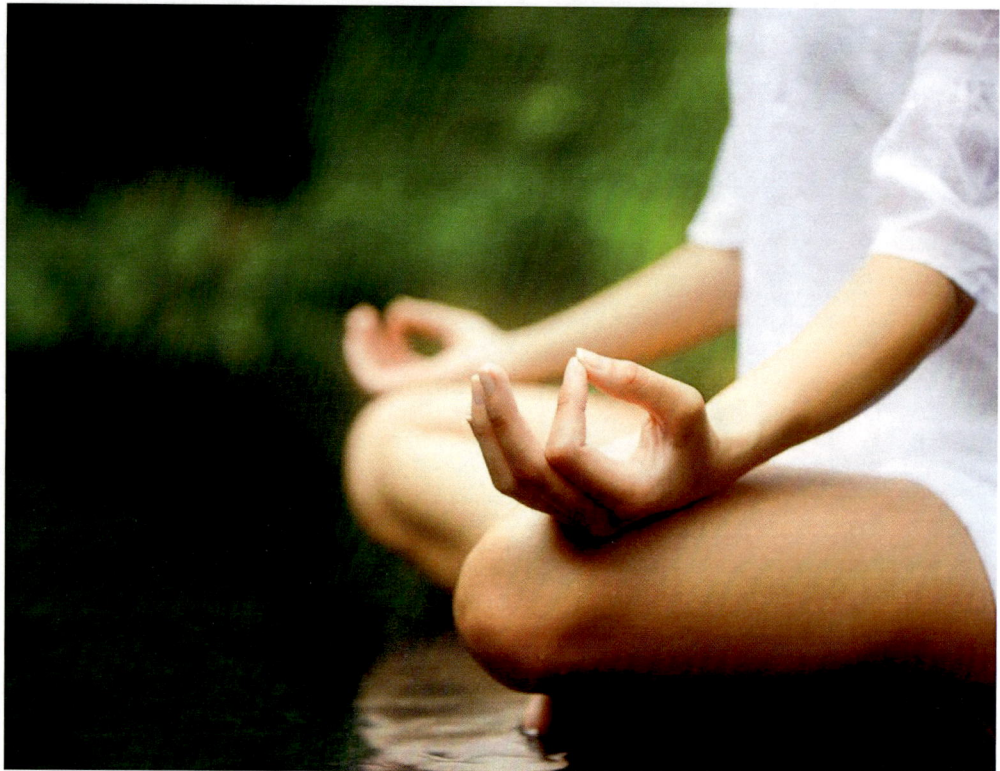

At the 5-week checkup with Dr. John Zurasky, it continued to be a high-five celebration with the recovery moving forward rapidly. Both my cognitive and motor skills still continued to move on a faster trajectory than expected, and my body began releasing the built-up fluids, so now I was down 45+ lbs and it was decided I'd be moving from 6 medications to 1, yes, down to 1 on the 1st visit! It was obvious that the **Recovery Plan** I had created was WORKING! Absolutely working. So, it was recommended to keep doing more of the same with a request to remember to rest and give myself time to fully heal. Close to that time in the conversation I told Dr.

Zurasky about my new immediate goal – Run a 5K that winter (slow and steady with no walking) return back to Marylhurst and begin working on my last 3 courses, be trusted to drive alone again, and of course, to smile and wink at will.    ;)

After continuing forward I was focused on gaining my complete independence back with the main focus of **GO**! And be **Grateful**!

The next appointment in 3 weeks was an additional surprise, the last medication also ceased and now I was up to 15 minutes of running, after 30 minutes of walking, and had made a promise with the nurse to try a Zumba class before my next appointment. Deal**!**  It was time to find **THE** race and detox with juicing.

**Reason for Living**:  Goals to support and accomplish – Still in love with life!

After a series of hearing tests with Dr. Hodgson it was determined that I would be stabilizing at 40% hearing in the right ear with constant tinnitus.  Although there were more options for additional treatments that would include more insertions or invasive techniques, I declined and told him I'd turn the ringing into backup music with a song that I could loop into my imagination, and continue to use the hearing loss as an aid for the times/people you actually don't want to hear, and now I can coyly do so by simply turning my heading slightly and rubbing that area right in front of my left ear that blocks sound.  We both started laughing.  I simply was done with "treatments" and in quite a celebration mode that of all of the scenarios I could've been faced with, I was left with a new privacy technique and backup mental music.  So be it.

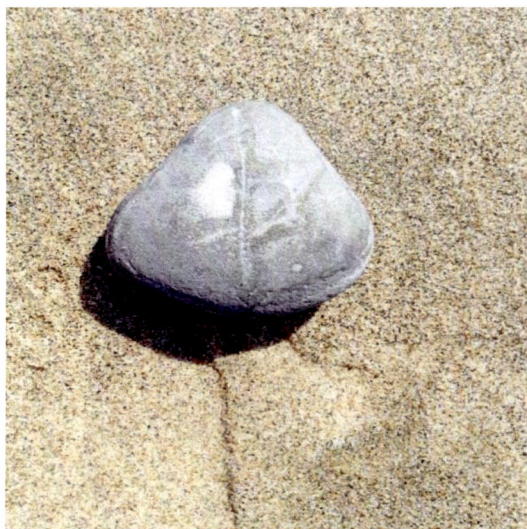

# The 5K Fort Vancouver Run on March 4th, 2012

## Mission Accomplished!

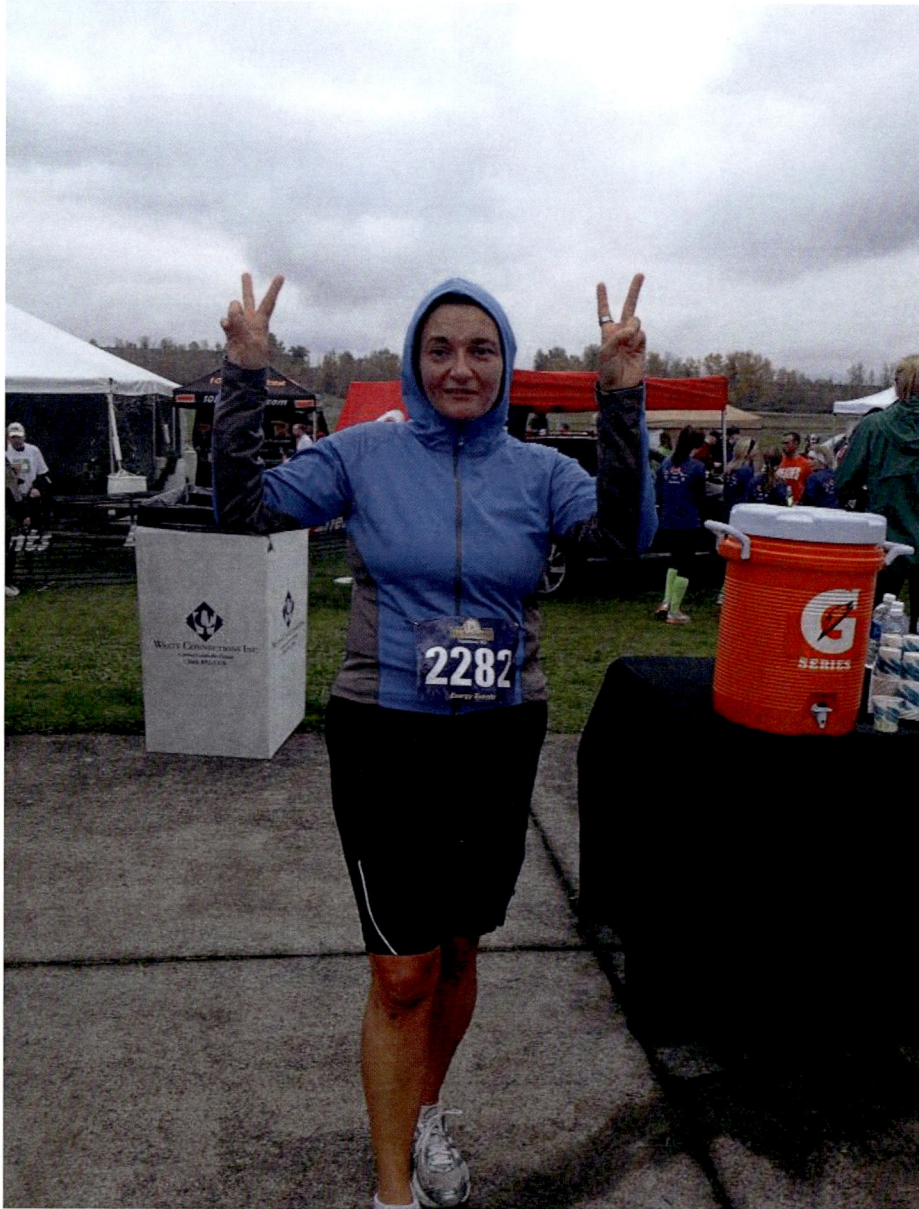

The following week I made a surprise visit to Providence ICU and the recovery unit with hugs, updates about the race, and thank you cards for all of my nurses. I wanted to get the opportunity to see them again and let them know that they were always appreciated and thought of. Your contribution makes a difference!

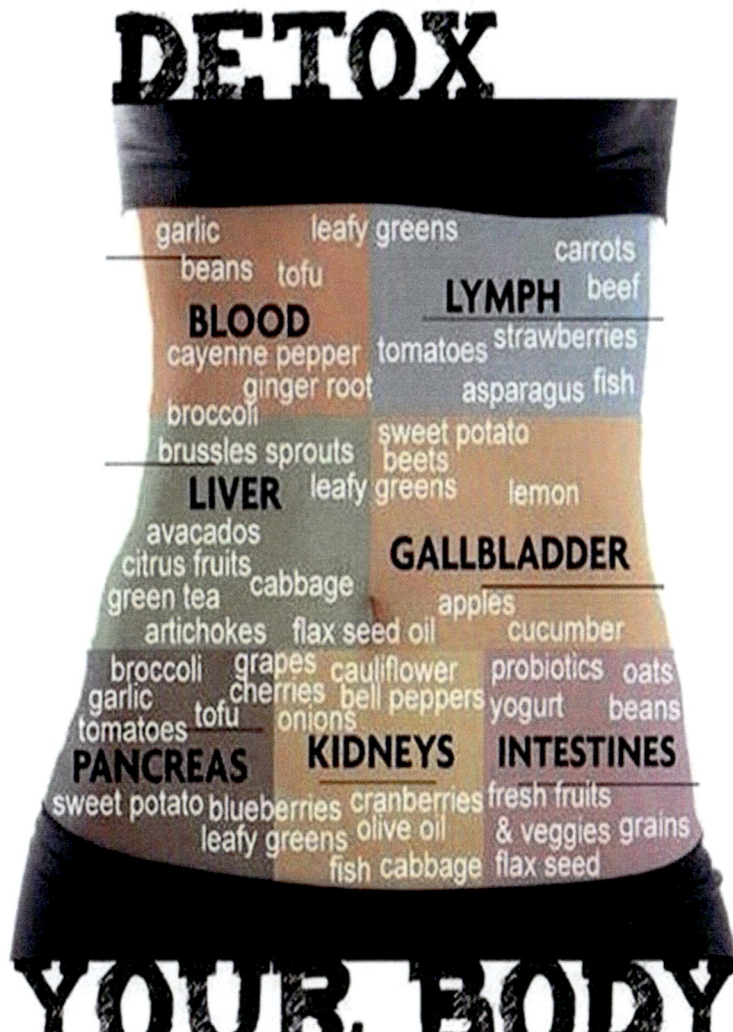

DETOX

garlic  leafy greens  carrots beef
beans  tofu
**LYMPH**
**BLOOD**
cayenne pepper  tomatoes  strawberries
ginger root  asparagus  fish
broccoli
brussles sprouts  sweet potato
beets
**LIVER**  leafy greens  lemon
avacados
citrus fruits  **GALLBLADDER**
green tea  cabbage
artichokes  flax seed oil  apples
cucumber
broccoli  grapes  cauliflower  probiotics  oats
garlic  cherries  bell peppers  yogurt  beans
tomatoes  tofu  onions
**PANCREAS**  **KIDNEYS**  **INTESTINES**
sweet potato  blueberries  cranberries  fresh fruits
leafy greens  olive oil  & veggies  grains
fish  cabbage  flax seed

YOUR BODY

Although I had yearly went on a 100% raw diet for 30 days and occasionally juiced, I began intensively researching the positive effects of temporarily moving onto a 100% juicing diet for a month, to clear my system and organs of the massive of amounts of medication that was pumped into my system, as well as fill it with massive amounts of supportive minerals, enzymes, and vitamins to help boost cellular repair and my immune system.  So, with probiotics added, I moved forward with this process.  The probiotics I chose to stay on for 2 more additional months. It's strongly recommended to research the benefits of both.  Share your thoughts and research results with me on *GetBackUP-Book.com*.

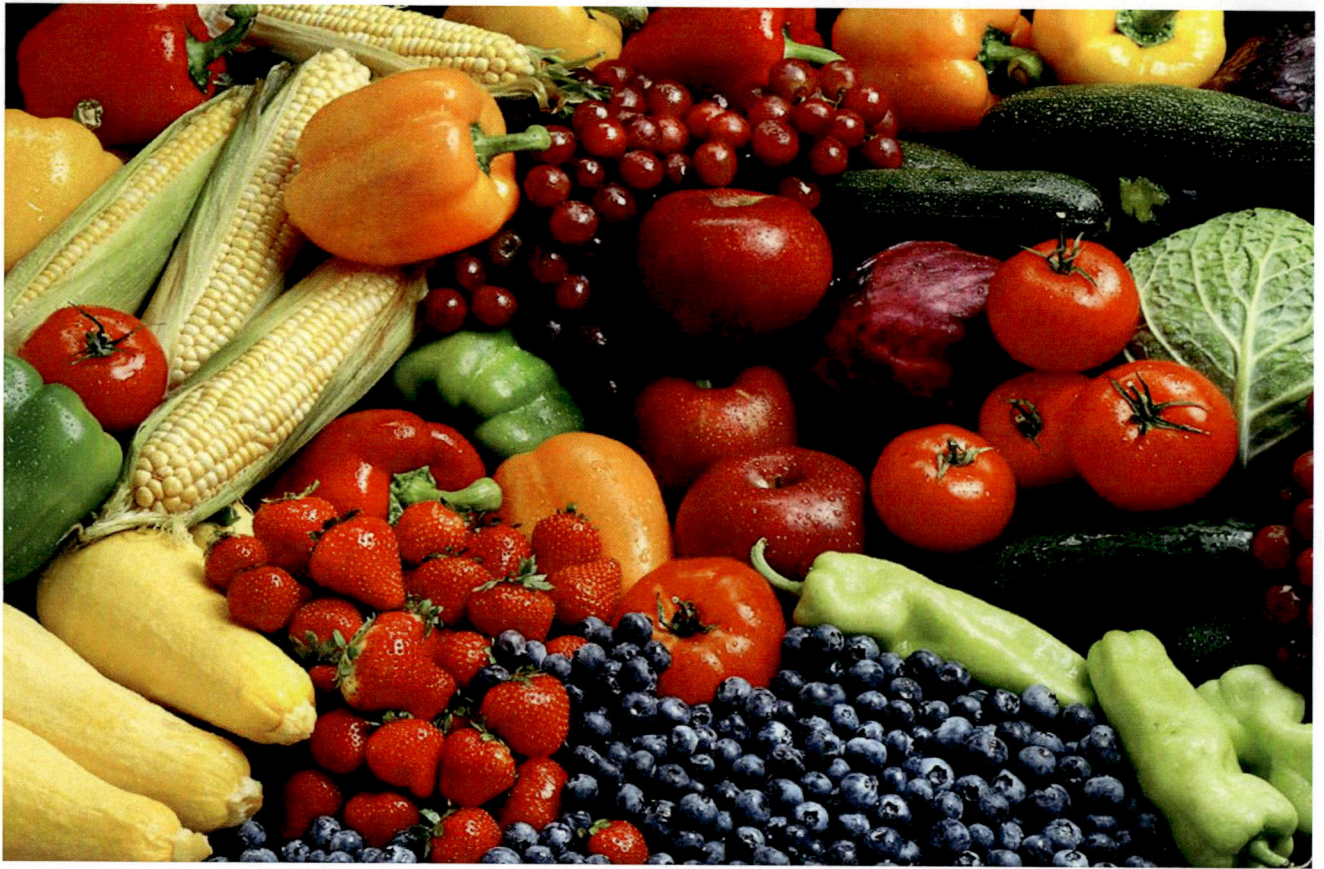

**Favorite Juice combos using The Bullet:**

- 1 Red beet, 1 lemon, 1 inch of ginger, 1 apple & kale.
- 3 Roma tomatoes, ½ red onion, clove of garlic, handful of basil.
- ½ cup of 6 hr. soaked raw cashews, 2 ears of corn kernels, stem of dill, 1 anaheim pepper, 1 clove of garlic, one stem of celery & basil.
- ½ Avocado, 1 cup of spinach, ½ cup of kale, ½ cup of pineapple.
- ½ Avocado, 1 cup of spinach, ½ cup of kale, handful of parsley, ½ lemon and a ¼ cup of fruit.
- 1 Pink grapefruit, 1 cup of kale, 1 inch of ginger, and 1 peach.
- 2 Large carrots, 1/2 fennel bulb, 2 green apples, 1 lemon, cayenne.
- 2 cups spinach or Kale, 1 orange, ½ lemon, 5 mint leafs
  Share your recipes with me  at **GetBackUP-Book.com**  **and https://www.facebook.com/getbackup2015.**

# List your Favorite Juice and Salad Recipes

# Book & Movie Recommendations

## (All videos can be found on Netflix)

Beautiful Truth (2008) – Video

The Science of Healing (2009) – Video

http://www.thehappymovie.com (2011) - Video

Fat, Sick, and Nearly Dead (2010) – Video

Gerson Miracle (2008) – Video

Food Fight (2012) – Video

Forks over Knives (2011) – Video

Chew on This (2012) – TEDtalks video

Dying to have known (2006) – Video

The Power of Habit: Why We Do What We Do in Life and Business (2006)–Author: Charles Duhigg – Ref. Virag Tunya

Botany of Desire (2001): Author: Michael Pollan

Future Diary (1989) –Author: Mark Victor Hansen

The Book Beyond Words – How the Soul Speaks (2012).  Author Paul NewHam

Raw Food – Real Word (2005).  Author:  Matthew Kenney and Sarma Melngailis

The Oh She Glows Cookbook – Over 100 Vegan Recipes To Glow From The Inside Out. (2014) Author: Angela Liddon – Ref. Virag Tunya

RAW & SIMPLE – EAT WELL AND LIVE RADIANTLY (2013). Author: Judita Wignall

A Symphony in the Brain (2008) Author: Jim Robbins – Ref. Dr. Noel

The Healing Power of Neurofeedback (2006) Author: Stephen Larsen – Ref. Dr. Noel

Restoring the Brain (2015) ed. Author: Hanno Kirk, PhD, LCSW  -  Ref. Dr. Noel

Share your recommendation with me at  *GetBackUP-Book.com and https://www.facebook.com/getbackup2015.*

# Recommended Medical Journals

1. AAPD - Association for Applied Psychophysiology and Biofeedback.  Article: Mind Body Medicine, Evidence-Based Medicine, Clinical Psychophysiology, and Integrative Medicine - 2011  http://www.aapb.org/i4a/pages/index.cfm?pageID=3386

2. National Center for Biotechnology Center - 2010
   Article: Top-Down and Bottom-Up Mechanisms in Mind-Body Medicine: Development of an Integrative Framework for Psychophysiological Research
   http://www.ncbi.nlm.nih.gov/pmc/articles/PMC2818254/

3. National Institutes of Health - 2005
   Article: Barriers to the Integration of Mind-Body Medicine: Perceptions of Physicians, Residents, and Medical Students
   http://www.explorejournal.com/article/S1550-8307(05)00205-3/references

4. University of Maryland Medical Center (UMMC) - 2015
   Article: Yoga – 2015
   https://umm.edu/health/medical/altmed/treatment/yoga

5. National Center for Complementary and Integrative Health (NCCIH) – 2013
   Article: Yoga for Health
   https://nccih.nih.gov/health/yoga/introduction.htm

6. ResearchGate
   A Journal of Positive Psychology – 2014
   http://www.researchgate.net/journal/1743-9760_The_Journal_of_Positive_Psychology

7. Empowered Patient Journal – 2015. Free Patient Journal Download towards the middle of the page. A Companion Journal for the Hospital Guide For Patients and Families http://empoweredpatientcoalition.org/patient-education/

8. Journal of Medical Ethics – 2002. Journal: Is there an advocate in the house? The role of health care professionals in patient advocacy. http://jme.bmj.com/content/28/1/37.full

9. Health Education Research - 2001 - Journal: Empowering counseling—a case study: nurse–patient encounter in a hospital http://her.oxfordjournals.org/content/16/2/227.full

10. Medstar Washington Hospital Center - 2015. The Empoweresd Patient – Journal: Your role in ensuring a safe and positive experience in the hospital. http://www.medstarwashington.org/for-patients/patients-and-visitors/patient-information/the-empowered-patient/#q={}.

11. International Society of Neurofeedback and Research 2015 - Journal: NeuroRegulation. http://www.neuroregulation.org/  - *Ref. Dr. Noel*

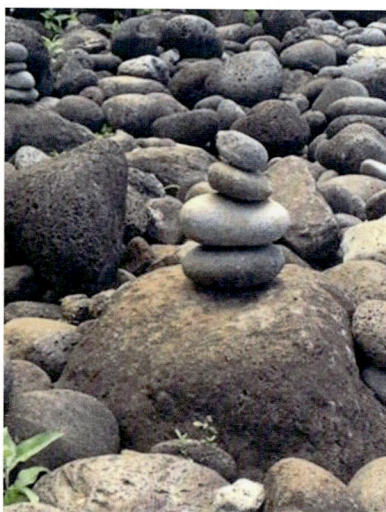

# The Role of the Patient Advocate - National Patient Safety Foundation

"Illness is a stressful time for patients as well as for their families. The best-laid plans can go awry, judgment is impaired, and put simply, you are not at your best when you are sick. Patients need someone who can look out for their best interests and help navigate the confusing healthcare system – in other words, an advocate.

## What is a patient advocate?

An advocate is a "supporter, believer, sponsor, promoter, campaigner, backer, or spokesperson." It is important to consider all of these aspects when choosing an advocate for yourself or someone in your family. An effective advocate is someone you trust who is willing to act on your behalf as well as someone who can work well with other members of your healthcare team such as your doctors and nurses.

An advocate may be a member of your family, such as a spouse, a child, another family member, or a close friend. Another type of advocate is a professional advocate. Hospitals usually have professionals who play this role called Patient Representatives or Patient Advocates. Social workers, nurses and chaplains may also fill this role. These advocates can often be very helpful in cutting through red tape. It is helpful to find out if your hospital has professional advocates available, and how they may be able to help you.

## Using an advocate – getting started

Select a person you can communicate with and that you trust. It's important to pick someone who is assertive and who has good communication skills. Make sure that the person you select is willing and able to be the type of advocate that you need.

 Decide what you want help with and what you want to handle on your own. For example, you may want help with:

- Clarifying your options for hospitals, doctors, diagnostic tests and procedures or treatment choices.

- Getting information or asking specific questions

- Writing down information that you receive from your caregivers, as well as any questions that you may have.

- Assuring that your wishes are carried out when you may not be able to do that by yourself.

 Decide if you would like your advocate to accompany you to schedule your tests, appointments, treatments and procedures. If so, insist that your doctor and other caregivers allow this.

• Be very clear with your advocate about what you would like them to know and be involved in

Treatment decisions? Any change in your condition? Test results? Keeping track of medications?

Let your physician and those caring for you know who your advocate is and how you want them involved in your care

Arrange for your designated advocate to be the spokesperson for the rest of your family and make sure your other family members know this. This will provide a consistent communication link for your caregivers and can help to minimize confusion and misunderstandings within your family.

Make sure your doctor and nurses have your advocate's phone number and make sure your advocate has the numbers for your providers, hospital, and pharmacy, as well as anyone else you may want to contact in the case of an emergency.

from: **National Patient Safety Foundation**
**132 Mass MoCA Way, North Adams, MA 01247**
**(413) 663-8900 www.npsf.org © 2003-2008**

# More Recommendations

Hospital Impact – Dissecting the Role of the Patient Advocate. http://www.hospitalimpact.org/index.php/2010/12/22/patient_advocates_guide_patients_through

National Support Groups – Peer/Community Support to help aid in their recovery. http://www.mentalhealthamerica.net/find-support-groups

US Health Department of Health & Human Services – Civil Rights http://www.hhs.gov/ocr/civilrights/resources/specialtopics/hospitalcommunication/lawsandregulations.html

Importance  for requesting an Advance Directive doc. from your hospital - Create a Living Will and an Advance Directive. http://www.patientsrightscouncil.org/site/advance-directives-definitions

Family Caregiver Alliance – National Center on Caregiving Hospital Discharge Planning: A Guide for Families and Caregivers https://caregiver.org/hospital-discharge-planning-guide-families-and-caregivers

Psychology Today – What is your Life Purpose https://www.psychologytoday.com/blog/prescriptions-life/201311/helping-you-find-your-life-purpose

The Two-Minute Defining Moment - http://www.huffingtonpost.com/william-horden/near-death-stories_b_2214176.html

*"Having a purpose is the difference between making a living and making a life."* ~ Tom Thiss

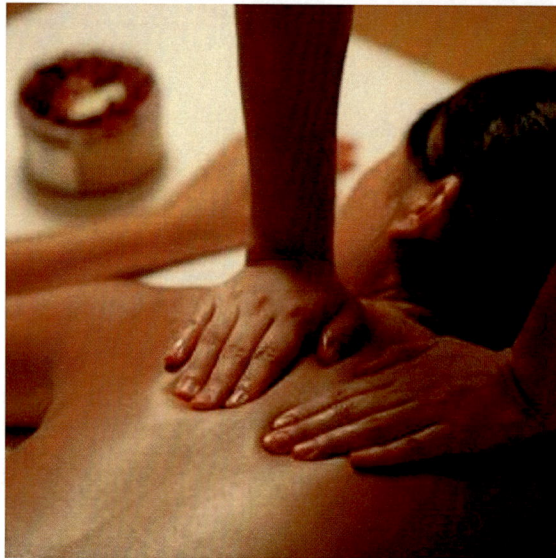

## Caretakers' Healing

Being the primary caretaker is tough. Many that experience intense emergency scenarios and long-term caretaking also experience **PSD (Post Stress Disorder)**. Remember to ask for assistance/ counseling as needed, seek out good nutrition, good health care, rest, massage, time alone, time for exercise, time for relaxation, and time for play.

Taking care of oneself is part of a Caretaker's job. The job is difficult and taxing, both physically and emotionally. It takes time to heal separately and together. It would be wise for insurance providers to add additional preventative care benefits/education for caretakers opposed to absorbing the larger mental and physical issues/costs that can occur from **not.**

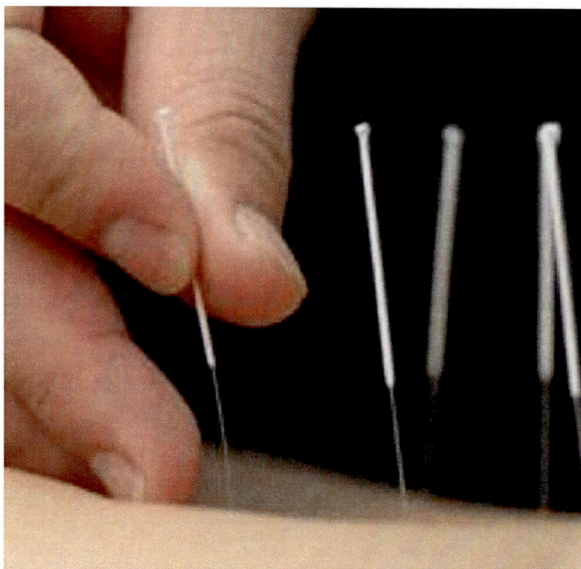

For me to graduate with my class in **September** 2012 I would have to take another leap of faith and return back to the Master's program in **March**, while taking the summer to complete the thesis. After registering for my courses I received a surprise call from my counselor that left me utterly speechless, **Marylhurst University** called to inform me that they wanted to scholarship my thesis course, as they were grateful that I survived my near-death experience, and was proud that I was an honor roll student; while requesting a graduation video interview.

## God, thank you. Thank you. Thank you!

It was in these moments it just solidified my deep passion to continue volunteering and patiently navigate all professional waters until I could fully integrate, and work with a dynamic medical institution or social organization full-time – permanently. Until such time the innovative tech/ engineering/ marketing world continued to be vast and intriguing.

I could feel that giving it my ALL professionally and personally, on every platform, was going to be extra exciting from this point forward, as I was pleasantly and hyper aware that every day is a GIFT. I see it clearly in Every smile. Every flower. Every sky I gaze at. And Every corner I turn.

### "Why am I here? What is my reason for living?"

With that deep commitment I also decided to move forward with having a Celtic symbol, representing the everlasting love of life, placed on my upper right arm. Although I knew I would have the task of professionally covering it in many chosen situations, I ultimately made the decision to continue to take actions that I drew strength from and have the tattoo placed on my upper right arm, staying near that right ear.

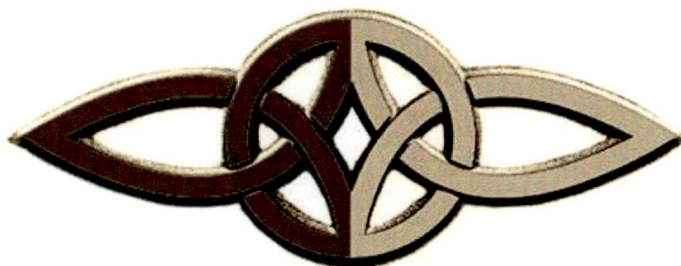

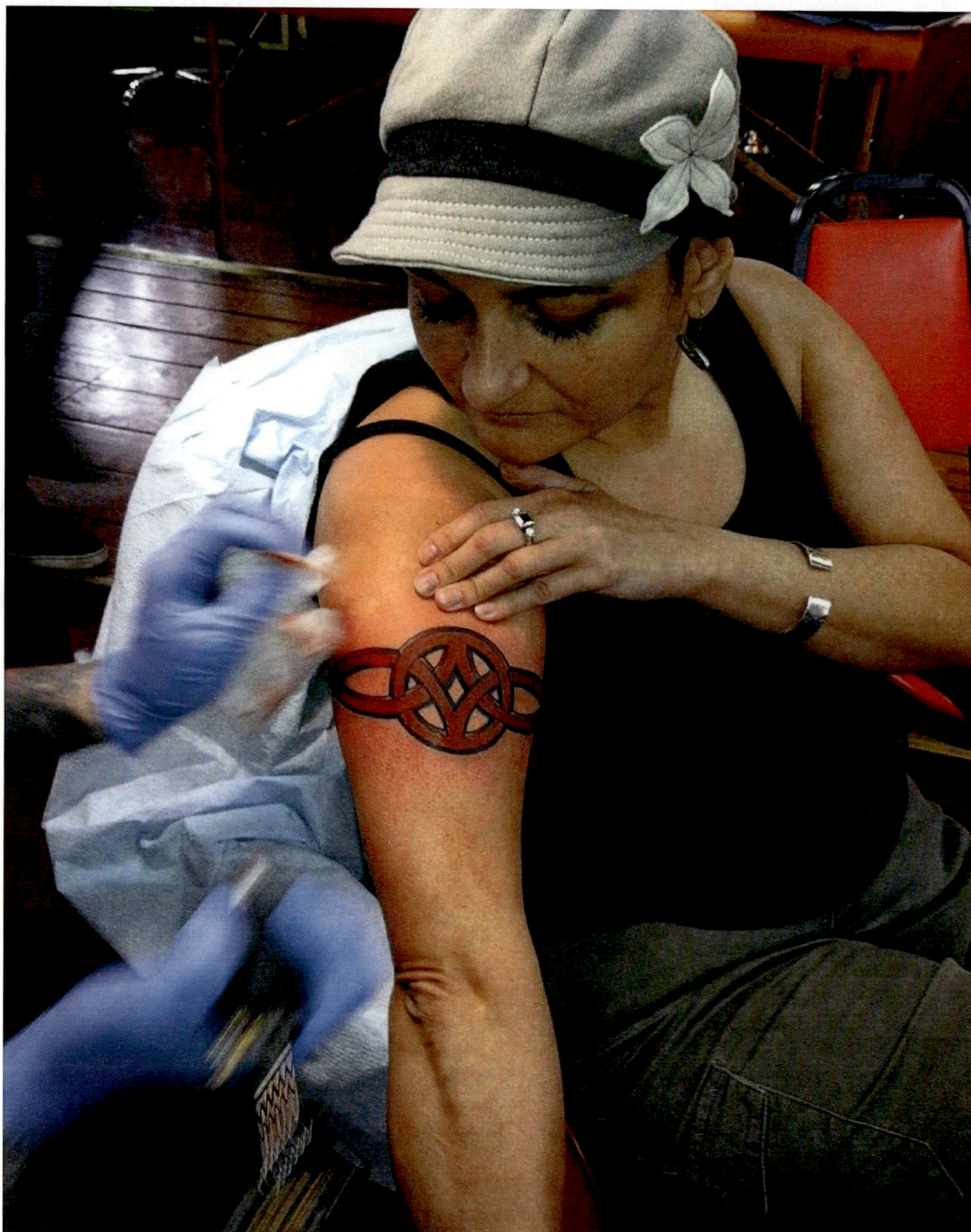

April 2012

Even with the ability to focus, accomplish, and always try to reach towards the positive, there were moments when I had fight not getting discouraged based on others fears and comments.  Although I was primarily surrounded with positive, caring, and devoted friends/family occasionally there were negative comments/persons that made occasional remarks that I had to shield my thoughts and emotions from, so it didn't alter my confidence and positive feelings.  Some included:

- "With your face being like that, you're going to have a hard time getting a job."
- "Just do anything, like work in a grocery store."
- "Wear more makeup."
- "I know you think it would be 'nice' to complete this degree but there's probably a good chance you may not be able too."
- "It's such a general Master's it may not really be all that helpful in your career."  (Note: The focus in the Master's is marketing which, besides business development and management, the majority of my entire career has been focused in. Huh?)
- "Eating like a goat isn't necessary.  I could NEVER do that."
- Etc.  Etc.  Etc.

**Advice**: Don't ever dummy down your capabilities because of someone else's vision and limitations.  Listen to your heart, your intuition, and your soul. If I had believed many portions of the decided reality, and a few negative opinions that had been thrown my way during this trauma, I wouldn't even be alive to share this story much less function near this level. I may even be going around in circles of victimhood and defeat. **Faith, hope, positivity, and empowerment is the key**. Make sure your inner voice is empowering you, not weakening you. I was fortunate that the majority of those around me, including **ALL** of the Providence staff, my physicians, and my nurses were the caring, supportive, empowering force I needed.  I was simply blessed and grateful as I sit here smiling and winking as I please.  Another finish line was coming.

**"The best moments usually occur when a person's body or mind is stretched to its limits in a voluntary effort to accomplish something difficult and worthwhile"**

— **Tal Ben-Shahar, Happier:** Learn the Secrets to Daily Joy and Lasting Fulfillment.

My grades for my last two courses were B's including my thesis which focused on The Optimum Strategies Non-Profits should use for maximum Business Development/Financial Management/Effective Marketing Growth.

# Michelle graduated with honors on September 4, 2012!!

## Graduating and celebrating the gift of LIFE with Family & Friends

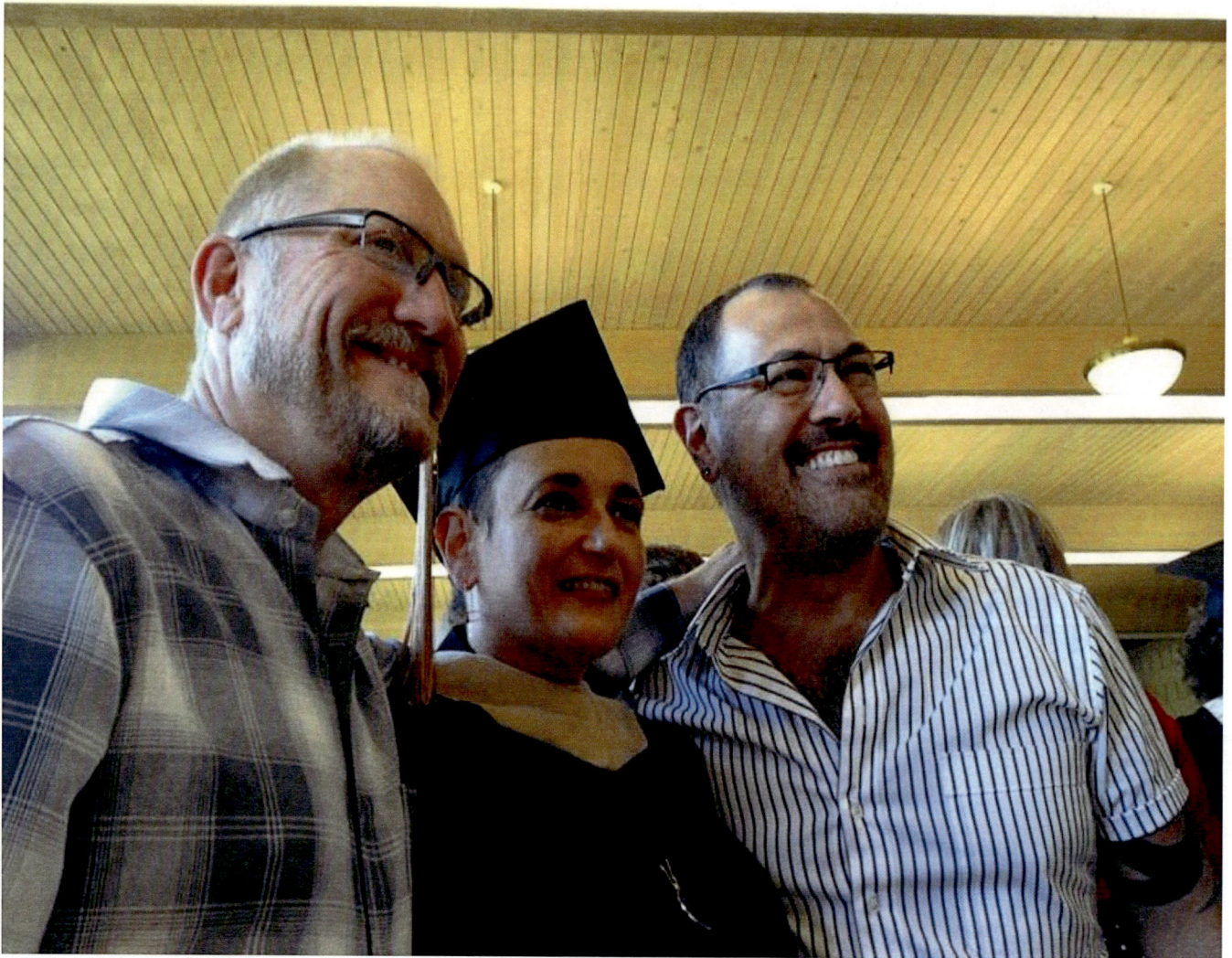

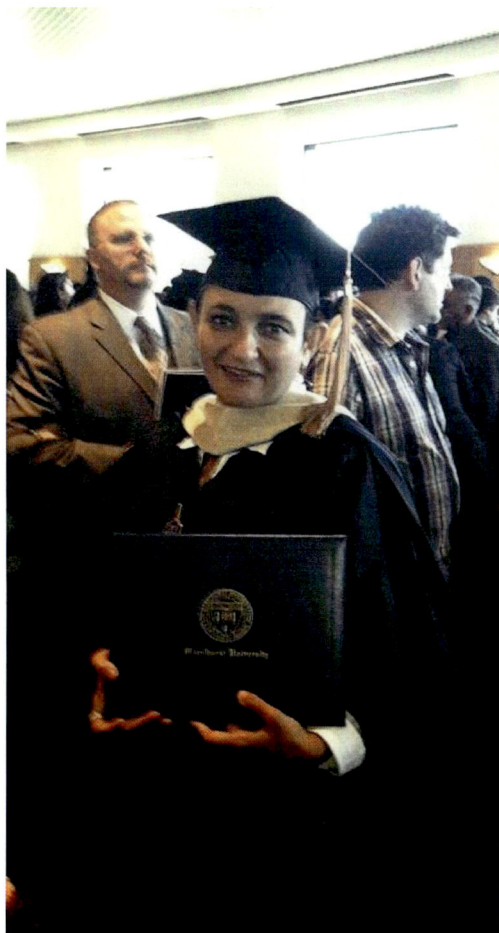

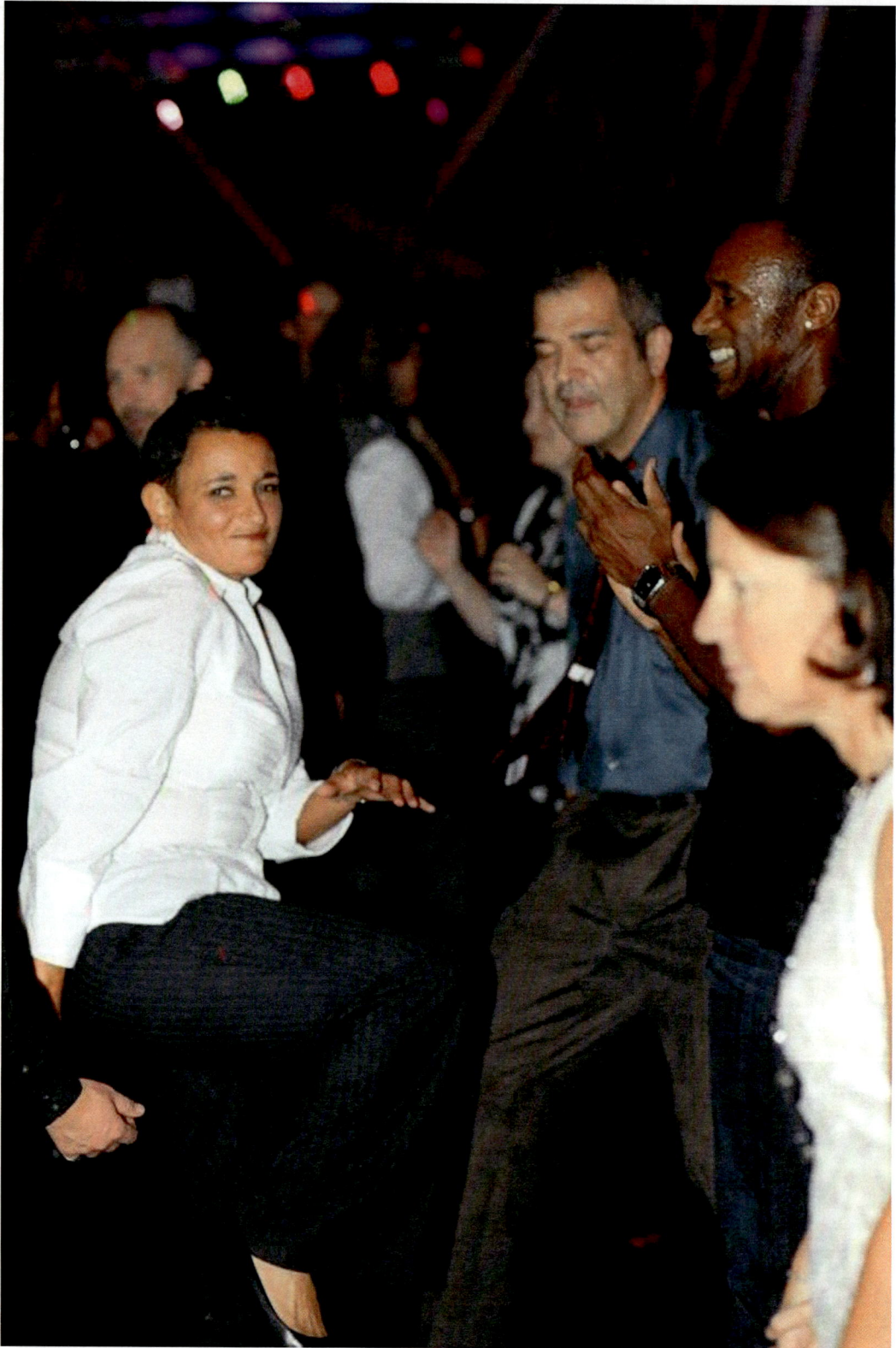

Let's celebrate it!

# List your TOP goals

_____
_____
_____
_____
_____
_____
_____

# List the things that bring you JOY

_____
_____
_____
_____
_____
_____
_____
_____

Share your thoughts with me  at  *GetBackUP-Book.com.*

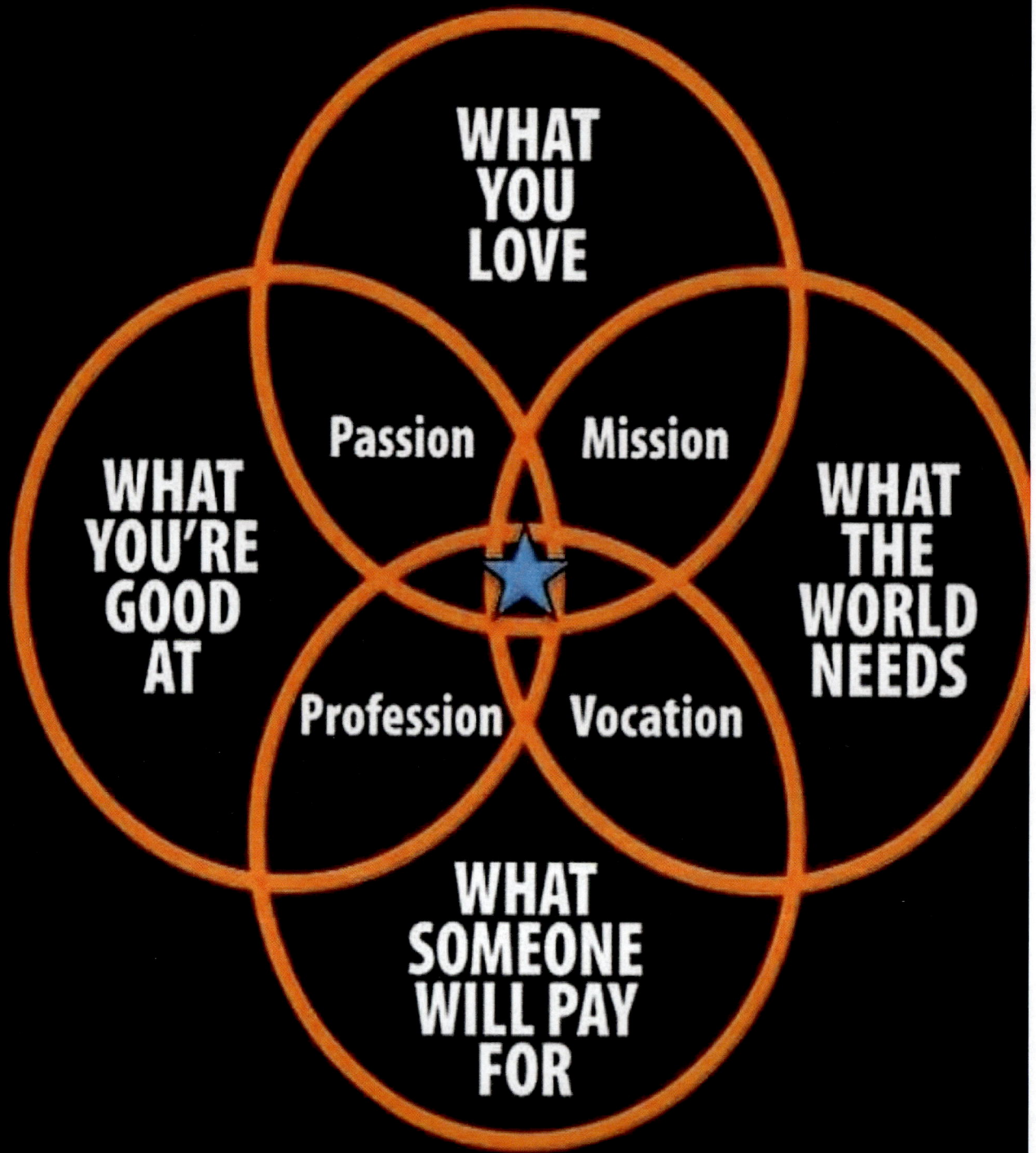

WHAT
YOU
LOVE

Passion     Mission

WHAT
YOU'RE
GOOD
AT

★

WHAT
THE
WORLD
NEEDS

Profession     Vocation

WHAT
SOMEONE
WILL PAY
FOR

★ = PURPOSE

# The First Portland 10K 2013 – Michelle & Virag

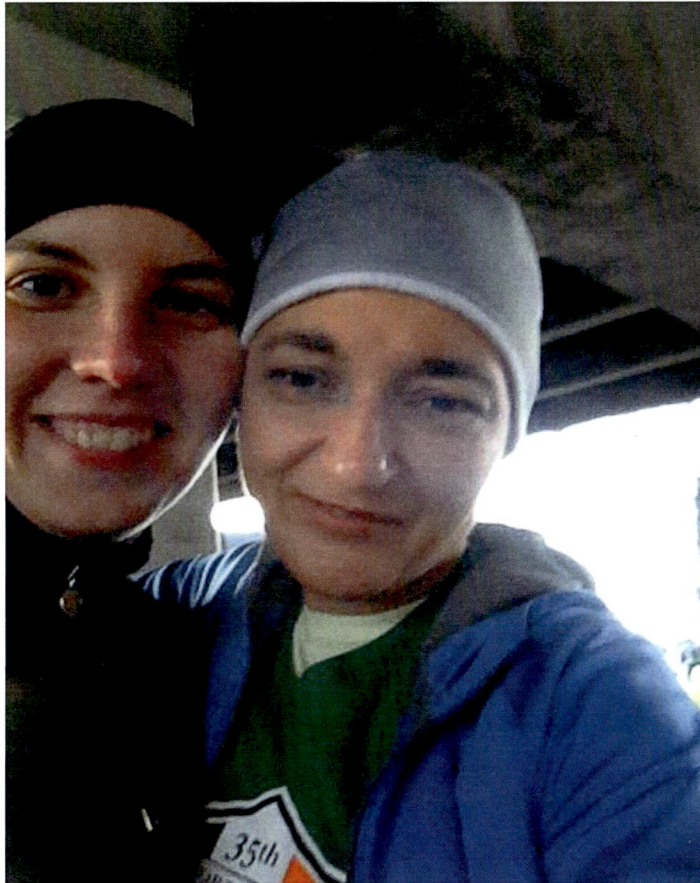

# The First Half-Marathon – Sauvie's Half on July 4th, 2014

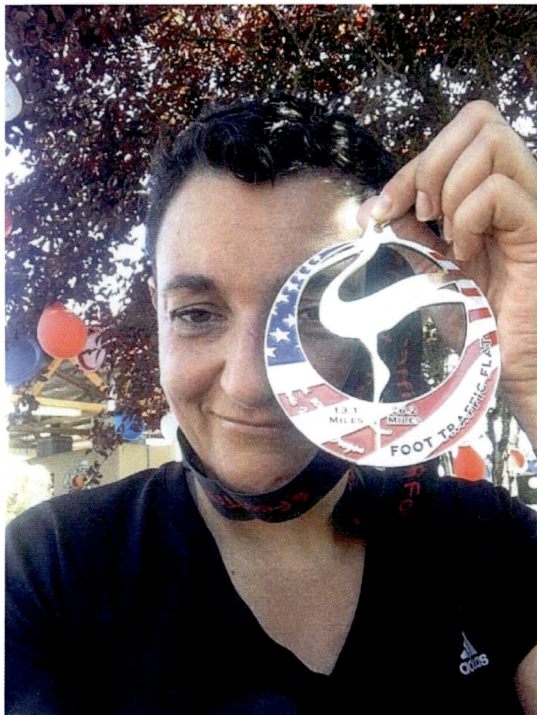

# The 2nd Half-Marathon – Kauai Half-Marathon on Labor Day 2014

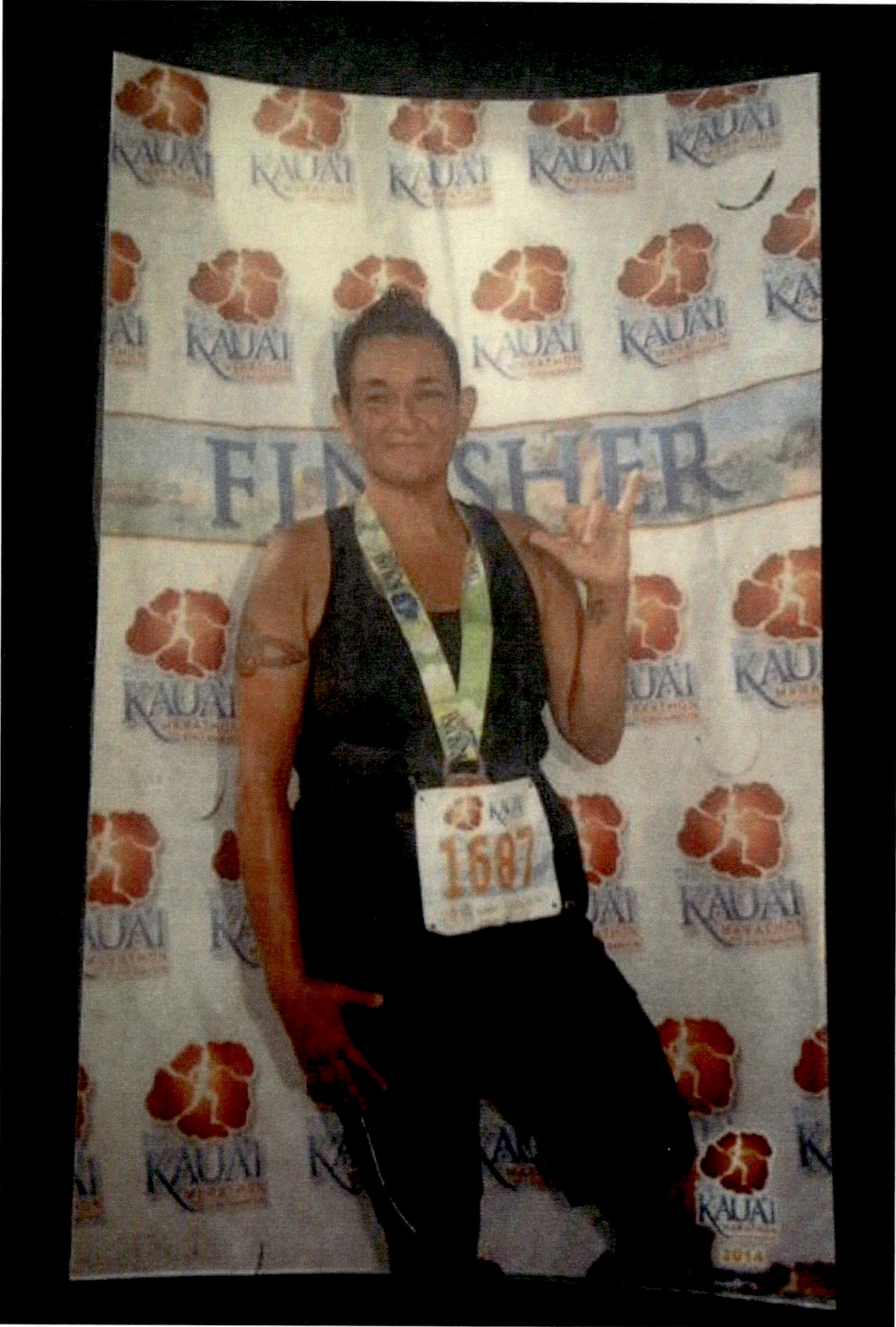

## *Memories & Reflections*

"No matter what kind of pain or condition you were in, you were always kind and said please and thank you to everyone. I would've turned into a monster." ~**Steven Nash**, Uncle

"It was a time that pulled people together for a common goal. It highlighted how some people handle stress, are patient, don't let go, while not getting attached to the outcome." ~**Lori Alfonso**, Friend

"It opened something in you. You are more joyful now, deeper thinking, more spiritual, more radiant, more grateful, and more passionate about life. ~**Angelina Swingle**, Sister

"Your experience reminded me of the ways we're thrown out into the sea and have to navigate the storms of life to survive, while holding on strong to our piers (family, friends, and community)... You inspire me; even talking on the phone with you gives me energy."
~**Larry Hanson**, Friend

"I can't put it into quotes how quickly life can change, so live it to the fullest and cherish it." ~**Berci Tunya**, Extended Family

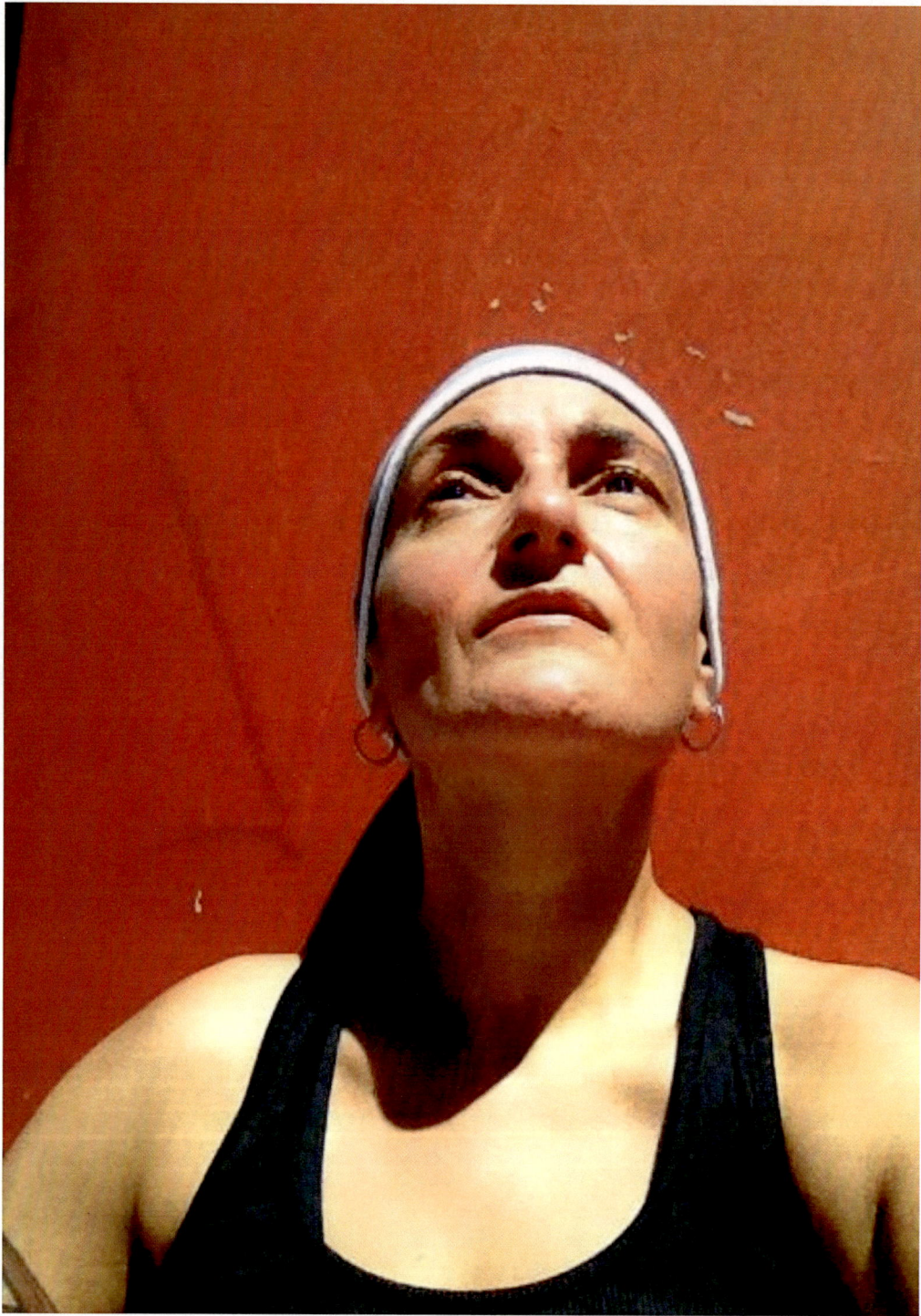

Trust the Voice within.

## Special thanks to:

Dr. Sterling Hodgson, Dr. John Zurasky, Dr. Lisa R. Yanase, Dr. Priscilla Le, Dr. Robert Lusk, Dr. Victoria Collins, Dr. Noel Thomas, David Tircuit LAc, Dianne Comins-Barrett, Yoga Instructor/Friend, Jennifer Fichter LMT, Sheila Resari LMT - *Thank you for helping save my amazing life and smile!*

**POEKOELAN TJIMINDIE TULEN** – Martial Arts

Extended Family - Berci & Virag Tunya.

Dan McCall and Rebecca Strack for giving me reiki.

Kerri & Larry Hanson, Stacey Dodson, Jeff Hurder, Arde Johnson, David Lefitz, Lori Alfonso, Zan Gibbs, and Janice Burger.

Youth mentors – Bob Havens, Sandy Meili, and Cindy Hooker.

To all who attended the special healing ceremony on my behalf at **The Movement Center and** all who prayed, meditated, and sent healing energy my way.

To my beautiful sister – Angelina Swingle.

Community and friends for surrounding me in positivity and support.

**Matt Hintzen**, today and every day.

**First Unitarian Church of Portland**

It was pleasure to speak at **Providence Hospital** in May 2013 - http://youtu.be/YFjfTvHKGGQ and again at the **Providence Foundation** dinner in 2014.

**Providence Mission**, *"We reveal God's love for all, especially the poor and vulnerable, through our compassionate service."*

Life

is not

measured

by the number of

breaths we take,

but by the

number of

moments

that take

our breath

away.

~Unknown

# Note to the reader:

I'm grateful to be able to share that this fortunate miracle occurred and after years of being private about its details, in certain spheres, I transformed and became inspired to create a site and write a book to help those seeking information, as well as offer another resource to explore, learn, and share from.

Often times we forget, in the fast motion of life, what may seem like common knowledge to us is in fact shared information and experience that took us years to become familiar and confident with. I was fortunate to enter into this period very healthy, strong, and had successfully explored many effective treatments prior so the network of quality health professionals was already established, as well as the other techniques I'd used. I also have health insurance that has good preventative benefits, which is highly recommended. I also recommend taking the time to build that network of professionals  and support groups so you always have a good base to lean into as needed and begin the use of **positive psychology**.

Many of the preventative health care plans include massage, acupuncture, naturopathic, and chiropractic care with established professionals in-network and with an affordable co-pay for 5-10 visits. Regardless if a health "problem" has occurred, it's wise to take advantage of the "preventative" treatments affordably, and use all of the visits yearly to continually keep balance, restore, ward-off, or work with the beginning of issues opposed to an escalated one. It also feels great to take good care.

It's also recommended to take a moment and find out where the gardening co-ops, fresh food programs, reduced organic grocers, health focused non-profits, community groups, your preferred hospital, and what the financial programs are around you so if resources are quickly reduced and an emergency occurs, you're prepared and have access to the support your needs. Please share your thoughts, resources, discoveries, and treatments with me and others at  **www.GetBackUP-Book.com**.

Take good care ~ *Michelle*

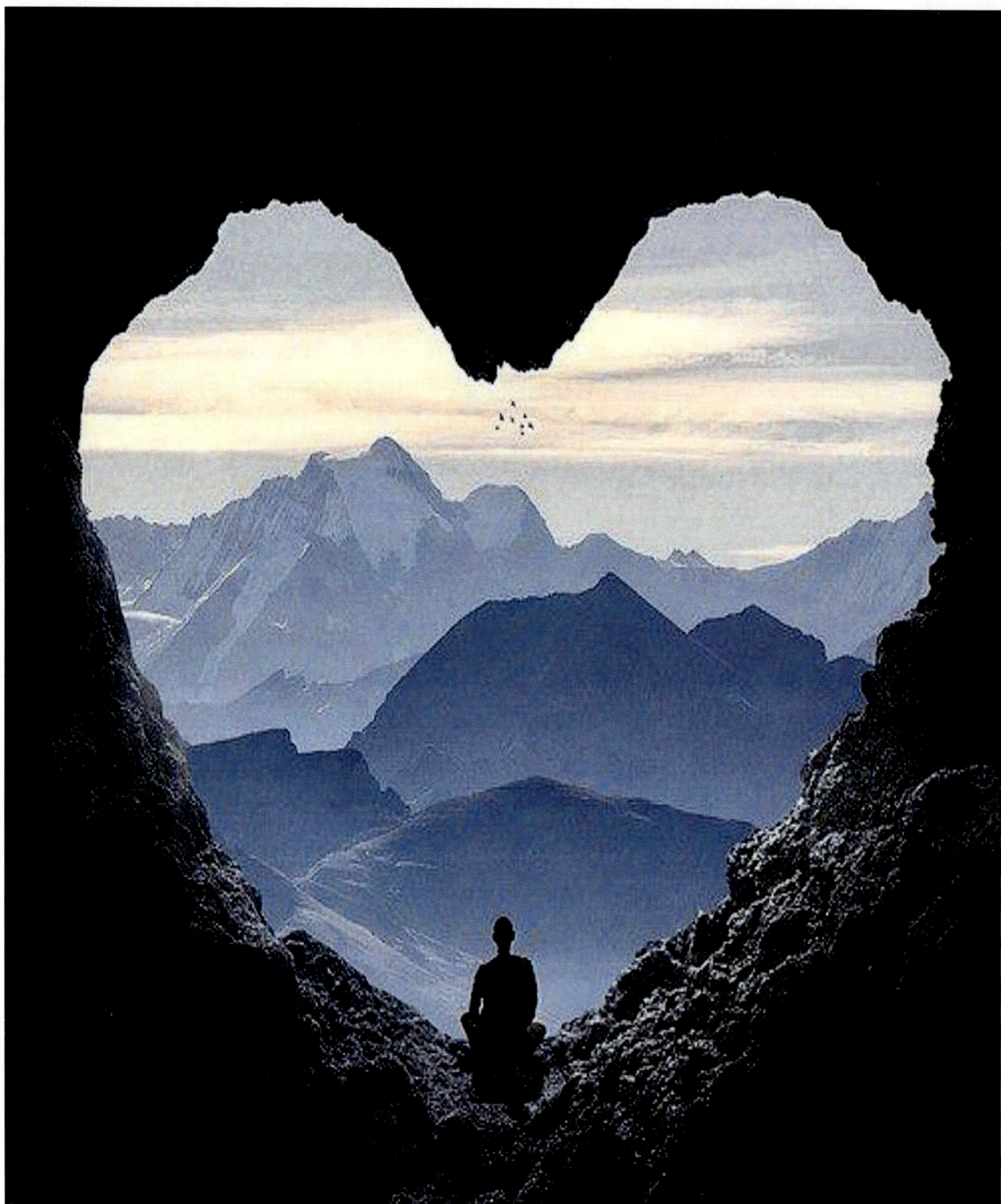

Namaste